Posture Pictures
Posture Assessment, Screenings, Marketing & Forms

DR. STEVEN WEINIGER
WITH RENEE NORTH, CPEP

Copyright 2011 © All rights reserved. Steven P. Weiniger DC
Posture Pictures: Posture Assessment, Screenings, Marketing & Forms
By Steven P. Weiniger DC, with Renée North, CPEP
Library of Congress Cataloging-in-Publication Data available on Request

ISBN-13 978-0-9797136-1-3
ISBN-10 0-9797136-1-7

Published by BodyZone Press
3000 Old Alabama Road
Suite 119-352
Alpharetta, Georgia USA 30022
770-922-0700
mail@bodyzone.com
www.BodyZone.com

Photography
Eric Bern Studio
Ed Wolkis Photography

Book design
Raheel Ahmed - For Emage Graphic Studio

Typeset
Absara, Flama, Gotham

Trademarks
BodyZone.com, the BodyZone.com logo, Move, Feel and Be Well, and StrongPosture™ and related trade dress are trademarks or registered trademarks of BodyZone INC or Steven P. Weiniger D.C. and may not be used without prior written permission. No part of this publication may be reproduced or transmitted in any form or by any means, electronic or mechanical, including photocopy, recording, or any information storage and retrieval system, without the prior written permission of the author.

DISCLAIMER: The information included in this publication is for educational purposes only and provided "AS IS" and you assume responsibility for determining the suitability of the information, and implementation of same, and for the results obtained. The user must assume the entire risk of using the information, including clinical appropriateness and accuracy of reports.

IN NO EVENT SHALL DR STEVEN WEINIGER, RENÉE NORTH, OR BODYZONE INC, ITS AFFILIATES, OR ITS SUPPLIERS, IF ANY, BE LIABLE FOR ANY CONSEQUENTIAL OR INCIDENTAL DAMAGES WHATSOEVER ARISING OUT OF THE USE OF OR INABILITY TO USE THE INFORMATION OR PROGRAM, EVEN IF THEY HAVE BEEN ADVISED OF THE POSSIBILITY OF SUCH DAMAGES. THEY SHALL NOT BE RESPONSIBLE OR LIABLE FOR LOST PROFITS OR REVENUES, OR FOR CONSEQUENTIAL, INCIDENTAL, DIRECT, INDIRECT, SPECIAL, PUNATIVE, OR OTHER DAMAGES OR FOR COSTS INCURRED AS A RESULT OF LOSS OF TIME, DATA OR USE OF THE INFORMATION, OR FROM ANY OTHER CAUSE INCLUDING, WITHOUT LIMITATION, LOSS OF BUSINESS PROFITS, BUSINESS INTERRUPTION, LOSS OF INFORMATION, OR OTHER PECUNIARY LOSS, PRODUCTS LIABILITY, CONTRACT OR TORT DAMAGES. LIABILITY SHALL NOT EXCEED THE ACTUAL PRICE PAID FOR THE INFORMATION OR LICENSE TO USE THE INFORMATION OR PROGRAM. BECAUSE SOME STATES/COUNTRIES DO NOT ALLOW THE EXCLUSION OR LIMITATION OF LIABILITY FOR CONSEQUENTIAL OR INCIDENTAL DAMAGES, THE ABOVE LIMITATION MAY NOT APPLY TO YOU.

This book is dedicated to the health, fitness and wellness professionals who make it their life's work to help others enjoy active, happy, healthy lives.

Special thanks to the Certified Posture Exercise Professional (CPEP) network for your ongoing support, ideas and inspiration.

Move, feel and be well.

Contents

Chapter One	Building Value	09
Chapter Two	Cameras and Software	17
Chapter Three	Posture Picture Assessment Protocols	23
Chapter Four	Posture Assessment Concepts	31
Chapter Five	Posture Assessment	37
Chapter Six	Communicating Posture Findings	69
Chapter Seven	Posture Screenings	75
Appendix A	Marketing Flyers	85
Appendix B	The Five Posture Principles	91
Appendix C	Posture Assessment Forms	101
Appendix D	Patient/Client Intake Form	103
Resources		105
About the Authors		115

CHAPTER ONE

Building Value

The future of healthcare will not look like the past. Like it or not, mounting financial pressure on our healthcare system will increasingly force people to pay for care out of pocket. With 77 million boomers approaching their elder years, this trend will continue to accelerate, and as a result the health and fitness industries will become more and more consumer oriented.

Health and wellness professionals can thrive in these changing times by providing services people value...and are willing to pay for out of pocket. Choice of care is driven by perceived value and cost, so it is imperative to increase perceived value, especially when personal pay economics are involved.

Multi-billion dollar pharmaceutical marketing campaigns exist to create value in the patient/consumer's mind, and creating value is also a path to success for practices focusing on posture. It's not just boomers, but anyone who wants to move well. Kids with backpacks, athletes seeking a performance edge, and desk bound

Relative Contributions to NHE By Source of Funds, 1999 to 2019 (in Billions)

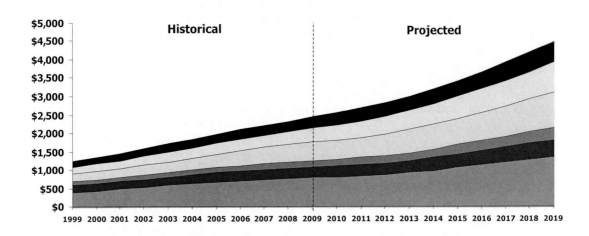

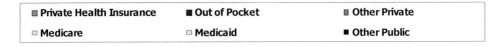

Note: First projected year is 2009.
Source: Centers for Medicare and Medicaid Services, Office of the Actuary, National Health Statistics Group, at http://www.cms.hhs.gov/NationalHealthExpendData/03_NationalHealthAccountsProjected.asp#TopOfPage (see Projected; NHE Historical and projections, 1965-2019, file nhe65-19.zip).

RelativeContributions to National Health Expense, 1999 to 2019 (in Billions)

computer jockeys are all increasingly receptive to posture based messages.

Creating posture consciousness, and then helping people strengthen posture, fills a niche which will continue to grow.[1]

Posture is How you Balance your Body

2nd Posture Principle

When I teach people about posture and exercises to strengthen posture, their eyes frequently light up as they ask about their body, their problems, and the role posture plays. Occasionally they pull their shoulders back and tell me they know they need to stand up straighter. When I ask why they don't, it usually comes down to "I forget about it" or "I can't". Either way, people "get" the importance of posture... especially the boomers who don't want to lose function as they age.

People's understanding of the connection between strong posture, good health and aging well is enhanced with visualizations to make this common-sense concept concrete.

Think of a winning athlete

    Is his posture strong and tall, or weak and slumped?

Think of an older person who is active and the way you want to be at 80...

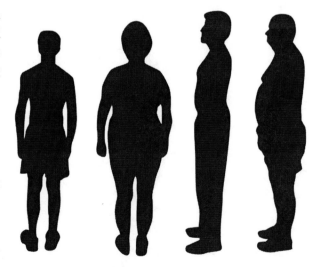

Who has Balanced Posture ?

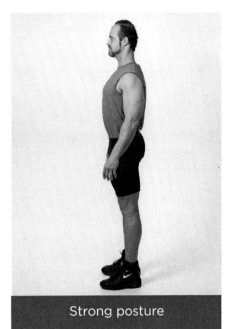
Strong posture

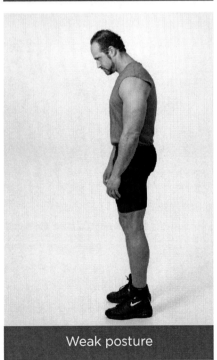
Weak posture

Is their posture erect or folding?

Now, think of an older person who isn't aging gracefully...

Are they standing tall, or are they hunched over, perhaps even using a cane or walker?

In our era of hyper-transparency not only must a marketing effort follow common sense, it must be scrupulously ethical and honest, eschewing misleading gimmicks and keeping patient benefit paramount. To be effective over the long term, efforts to create value must be in alignment with science, and able to withstand government regulations and the shining light of the internet, social media and ever multiplying blogs.

Posture is holistic and aligned with common sense and the evidence biased care model, as espoused in the book *How Doctors Think*[2]. First, biomechanically we stand and move with whole motions, not thinking about if our head is jutting forward or our knees turning in. Second, from a global health perspective, posture is a reflection of how well a body is working and how someone is feeling. A quick glance at body language tells us if someone is depressed (with their shoulders slumped), feeling down (and looking at the floor) or on top of the world (and standing tall).

Contemporary research demonstrates that posture truly provides a window to health, and suggests a path to improve health that people understand and will value, especially when they see and feel posture changes and understand how strengthening posture can truly make a positive difference in overall health.

According to the *Harvard Medical School Adviser*, "Research suggests that vertebral fractures have been overrated as a cause of height loss and hunching. Another big reason may simply be bad posture.[3]"

A 20 year University of London study looked at over 4,200 men aged 40-59 and found strong correlation between losing height and mortality. The authors speculated that slumping over postures caused a physical restriction of breathing which significantly increased risk of cardiovascular disease, stroke and respiratory mortality.[4]

Women with a jutting forward head posture were found to have almost half again the risk of dying during the course of one 4 year study.[5]

People with strong posture breathe better, look better and exercise more effectively,

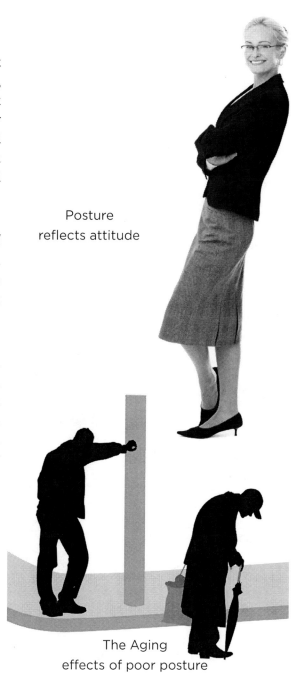

Posture reflects attitude

The Aging effects of poor posture

Screenings can find early posture problems

Posture Distortions can be improved.

all factors desired by patients and clients searching for ways to age well. The best way to create posture awareness, as well as a great first step in strengthening posture, is to simply take a posture picture.

Use the posture image to educate patients and clients about the difference between Weak Posture and Strong Posture, and as a tool to explain your findings and recommendations.

Comparison Posture Picture Reports can demonstrate changes and improvements after a course of treatment. In addition to creating a baseline for treatment plan follow-up, creating posture awareness can open the door for annual posture exams to observe and monitor posture changes over time.

Posture pictures create a marketing edge by showing people what they know and can relate to, and then helping them understand more about posture and biomechanics to their level of interest.

Recognize that even though you can get a lot of information about a body's biomechanics and function from a posture picture, from a marketing point of view you probably don't need or want to explain to a patient every detail.

You do need to show them enough to know and understand the importance of maintaining strong posture as they age in order to create and increase their understanding of posture and the value of your services.

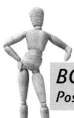

BONUS: *See Appendix A for Posture Analysis Marketing Flyers*

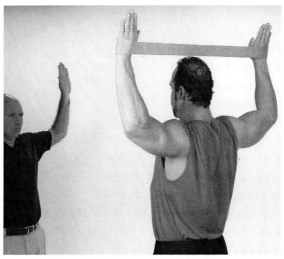

Focused Posture Exercise

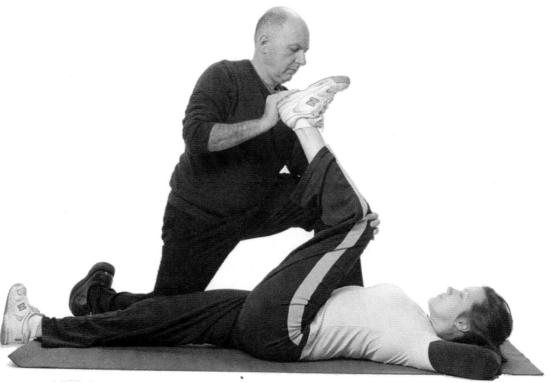

Postural muscle therapy

CHAPTER TWO

Cameras and Software

What do I need to take posture pictures?

A $20,000 software and video camera system has more features than a digital camera, but both can take a picture of posture. The question is - what are you going to do with it?

If research is your goal, you'll want a system which provides the highest possible standards of reproducibility. Factors as varied as maintaining an absolutely constant distance and squaring of camera, subject and background, floor surface, visual references in the background, lighting, operator training and a host of others must be controlled.

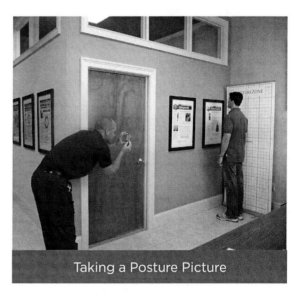
Taking a Posture Picture

In a rigorous research setting a more expensive system may be justified. However, for the majority of clinical or athletic assessments, a well-designed inexpensive

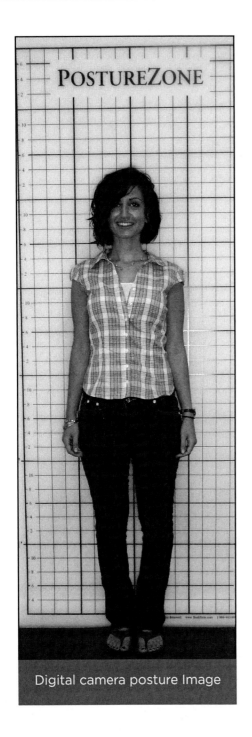

Digital camera posture Image

system will likely provide all the features and functionality you desire.

Ask yourself these two questions:

> Does the system show me what I need to see?

> Does the system show the patient / client what they need to see?

The line between what you need to see and what they need to see will be determined by the practitioner, technique and patient's desire to understand. In the following pages there is a lot of information, most of which is for you, and some of which is for the patient. We leave it to the clinician to decide what is relevant and what is secondary or incidental to the individual patient.

Unless a technique requires precise, x-ray correlated measurement for a clinical determination, most clinicians do not require the scientific precision of high end systems. In other words, each individual practitioner must assess the clinical level of accuracy they require.

On the other hand, what do patients / clients need to see? Images capable of creating value in the patient's eye can be taken with a digital camera and printer. Color is better, but black and white can also work extremely well.

Camera

A basic 5 megapixel digital camera is all you need. The ability to choose resolution and image size is helpful and a feature found on any modern camera, as well as being available on most webcams, smartphones or even inexpensive cellphones.

Getting Images from the Camera to the Computer

Technology keeps giving us more ways to import a picture to the computer.

Old School Technology

By Wire: Physically connect your camera to the computer, usually with a USB cable.

- Best for: Fixed location setups, usually in-office
- Disadvantage: Can be inflexible, and you have to deal with /bring a cable

By Card: Take the memory card or memory stick out of the camera, and put it in the computer. Card readers are built into many PCs, or USB readers are available for less than $15.

- Advantage: Easier to transfer photos / no cable needed
- Disadvantage: Keeping track of tiny memory cards.

New Technology

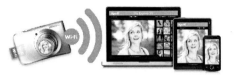

Eye-Fi Wireless SD Cards *(www.eye.fi)* - A memory card that makes your camera wireless. You take the picture and it is automatically saved to your computer.

    Advantage: Speed and flexibility

    Disadvantage: Cost (about $50) and setup (straightforward)

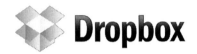

Internet Camera/Phone + DropBox - DropBox *(www.dropbox.com)* is a personal file folder that is hosted in the cloud of the web. If your camera has an internet connection (like iPhones or other smartphones) you can set up a free DropBox account, and save your photo to it. Your computer with access to the same account will be able to see and use the images.

    Advantage: Flexibility, remote access to images

    Disadvantage: Needs internet connection, variable (short) lag time for images to appear

Software

While some posture professionals invest in elaborate software and/or hardware systems, others merely take a picture, print it out, and then use a marker to draw gravity lines and demonstrate asymmetry to the patient.

However, if one of the goals of posture pictures is creating the perception of value, then a professional presentation showing the patient what they need to know is important. Many posture professionals use a posture assessment software program to generate a report for the patient.

These programs usually allow basic image editing, cropping, adjusting brightness for over and under-exposure, and other features including drawing lines and measure degrees of deviance from true vertical or horizontal. These are all valuable in demonstrating biomechanics and value to a patient.

However, be aware that programs with proprietary algorithms to rate the patient's "posture number" according to a "secret formula of ideal posture" will be viewed by patients (and other professionals) as a marketing driven gimmick.

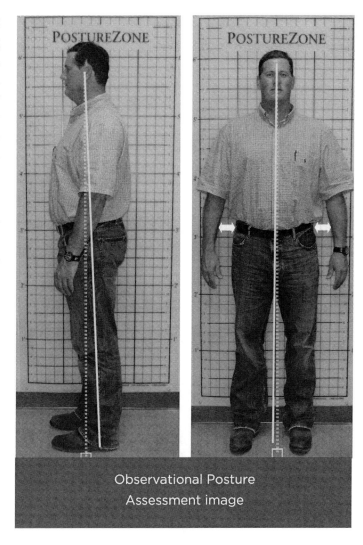

Observational Posture Assessment image

When choosing posture assessment software, be sure to ask:

- How much does it cost? (at the time of this printing most posture assessment programs range from $499 to $2000, with a couple in excess of $20,000)
- Is there a monthly or yearly maintenance fee?
- What is the cost for updates?
- Is there a cost or fee per report printed?
- Is the program web-based (connecting to the internet is an issue at some posture screening events held outside the office)
- How many computers can I install the program on? (most programs come with a single user license, meaning you can install on one office computer)
- How much does an additional user license cost? (plan to use the program on your office desktop computer, and on a laptop computer for community events)
- Does the vendor provide support? Is there an additional cost for support?

Posture assessment pictures are an excellent tool to begin a dialogue with a new or prospective patient or client. With the posture picture (or posture report) in hand you can use words to describe the biomechanics of posture, and then allow the picture, and later the comparison report, to speak for itself.

When it comes to posture assessment software, I lean towards a straightforward "just the facts" approach. For most practitioners, an inexpensive program that offers the basic image editing tools mentioned above, comparison reports, and allows you to perform a fast assessment will give you what you need for posture screenings, patient / client communications and documentation.

In our media drenched world, a posture report with simple lines to explain biomechanics, and then noting significant observations gives credibility, and credibility is essential in creating and building the perception of value.

CHAPTER THREE

Posture Picture Assessment Protocols

"Man will become better only when you make him see what he is like" - Anton Chekov

Taking clinical posture pictures requires consistent positioning. Especially when used for annual re-examinations, it is imperative to minimize image variation and distortion from camera and/or patient positioning & instruction. Depending upon the space available, your posture picture process must account for background, camera positioning, subject positioning and subject instructions.

Background

It's important to take posture pictures with the subject standing in front of a wall or background where true vertical and horizontal reference points are readily apparent. Floral wallpaper and outdoor sites with no background will result in images without useable references.

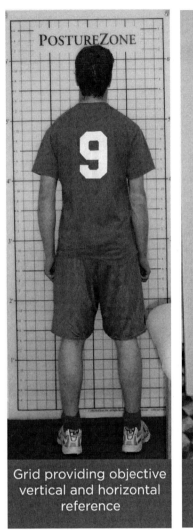
Grid providing objective vertical and horizontal reference

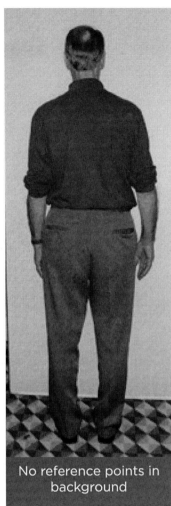
No reference points in background

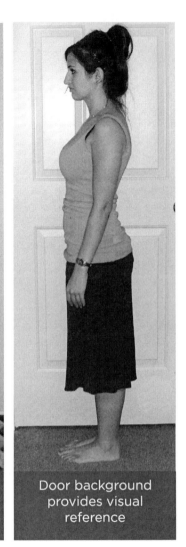
Door background provides visual reference

Are the shoulders level and the head tilted, or vice versa?

Posture grids provide consistent vertical and horizontal background reference points which makes clinical assessment easier and more accurate, as well as adding a strong professional touch. However, a door frame or a six panel door can suffice in a pinch for a visual vertical reference.

Many posture assessment software programs allow you to overlay a "digital grid" on top of the image. Using this feature to align the digital grid with a wall grid allows leveling of the image to near tripod accuracy.

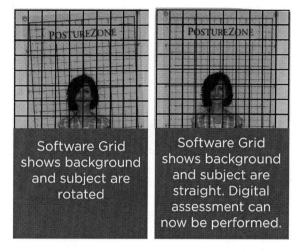

Software Grid shows background and subject are rotated

Software Grid shows background and subject are straight. Digital assessment can now be performed.

Camera Positioning

To minimize distortion the camera should be parallel to the background wall and the area evenly and well lighted. Hold the camera level with the ground (a tripod is helpful but not essential). Standardization for comparison reports can be achieved with a tripod or other device to fix the camera (ideal) or by placing a marker on the floor (a taped X) to indicate camera positioning.

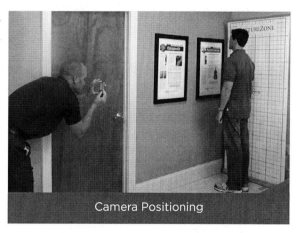

Camera Positioning

Distance to subject: We recommend 10 feet; however, it is important to maintain an adequate distance to fully visualize the subject in the camera view-finder.

Subject Positioning

Foot pads or other devices to tell people "how to stand" are not recommended. The goal of functional posture assessment is assessing what the individual internally thinks is "straight". Therefore, placing the feet symmetrically (but unnatural for the individual) will cause compensation as feet which "normally" evert are held straight and compensation then propagates up the kinetic chain of posture. If you want to indicate approximately where the subject should stand, a better option is an "X" taped on the floor.

Anatomical Markers: Consistently marking anatomic landmarks can significantly increase accuracy when drawing assessment lines. We suggest inexpensive ½ inch colored stickers, available at any office supply store.

Note: Be sure the subject cannot see their reflection in a mirror, glass picture frame or other reflective surface. People will subconsciously self-correct posture if a visual cue is available.

Subject Instructions

Tell the subject you are going to take a picture to study the biomechanics of their posture. Have the person stand in front of a reference wall facing you. I suggest taking the AP *(Front View)* image first, your subject will be able to see you, minimizing anxiety and promoting relaxed posture. Do not allow the subject to touch or lean against the wall.

We suggest training all staff members who take posture pictures to use the identical words to cue the subject to improve uniformity of images as well as to create a consistent, professional impression on the patient.

1. *"Stand comfortably and look straight ahead"* (If using a floor marker, add *"over the X"*)

Watch for a rigid military "at attention" posture (i.e. bilateral shoulder or abdominal tightening). Patients will try to assume a "good" posture, so in order to observe a true "resting posture" it is important not to coach the patient by asking them to "straighten up" what is misaligned.

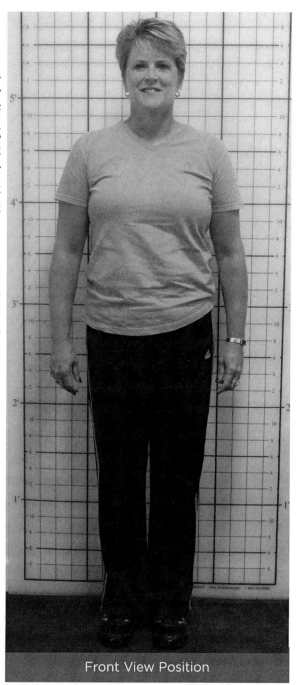

Front View Position

Posture Pictures

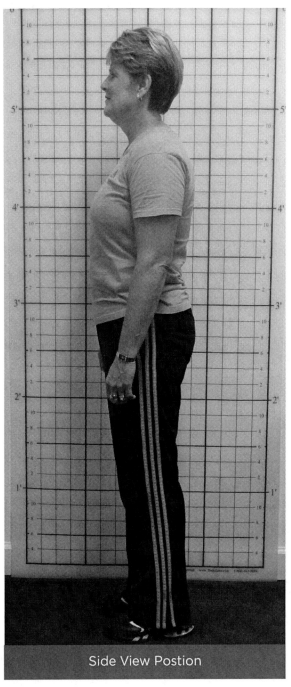

Side View Postion

The goal is to view their everyday posture, so if someone poses excessively or stands with neck muscles obviously quivering with effort, simply say *"Relax and stand comfortably."*

2. *"Take a deep breath in and let it out."*

Many people will hold their breath when you take the posture picture. Since the diaphragm is a core muscle, locking it can affect posture.

3. *"Stand straight and show me your best posture."*

When people see their posture distortions on a picture they frequently will say "I just wasn't standing straight". By instructing them to *"Stand straight and show me your best posture"* you help align their subjective perception with your objective observations.

> This creates an Aha! Moment when the patient / client sees their posture picture and realizes, *"I know you said to show you my best posture... I thought I was standing straight!"*

In addition, professionals teaching the StrongPosture™ exercise protocols use this "Best Posture" position as a baseline foundation for progressions to strengthen posture.

4. Take the picture and then say "Good."

Next, to take a Left Lateral *(Side View)* image say *"Now, turn and face the wall to your right."* and repeat steps 1 - 4.

It doesn't matter which side you use for the lateral view, but we strongly suggest you decide now whether you will have all subjects face the right or the left. Doing so now will ensure uniformity of before and after posture picture comparison reports.

Finally, take a PA *(Back View)* image by saying *"Now, turn and face the grid."* and repeat steps 1 - 4.

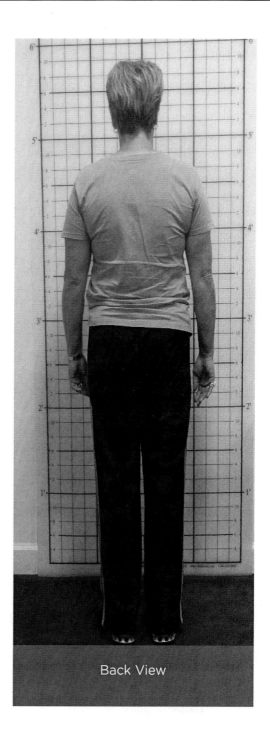

Back View

Note: Some people will stand in an obviously unnatural posture, often leaning back in an effort to simulate "good" posture. If so, reset their normal by instructing the subject to: "March in place for 3 steps," and then begin the cues again (1 – 4 above).

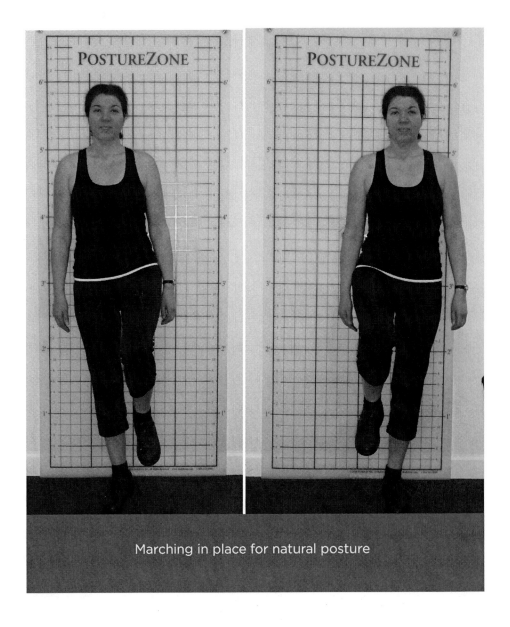

Marching in place for natural posture

CHAPTER FOUR

Posture Assessment Concepts

"If you are observant, you can see a lot." - Yogi Berra

Being judgmental is not always a bad thing. Some things are relative, and some are not. Mechanically speaking, there is good, strong posture and there is weak posture which is less mechanically effective. There are absolutes in bio-mechanics... Einstein's theory of relativity is not talking about poor posture. People understand the mechanical nature of posture, especially when explained using the Five Posture Principles.[6]

BONUS: See Appendix B for the 5 Posture Principles

Defining the one perfect and best way of assessing posture is beyond the scope of this manual. There are, however, simple and effective ways to observe the relationships between the four zones of posture, and use those observations to observationally benchmark both how the body is balancing in space, and note changes over time or with a course of therapy.

Professionals assessing posture range from doctors of chiropractic to physical therapists, from dentists to podiatrists, massage therapists to fitness trainers, as well as CPEPs Rolfers, Alexander and Feldenkrais practitioners, Pilates and yoga instructors and many other health, fitness and wellness professionals. These professionals use therapies which affect posture, ranging from the active to the passive, from osseous manipulation to soft tissue work using hands or elbows, instruments or machines.

Depending upon who is looking at posture, clinicians find significance in a variety of findings, according to their respective learnings. Some observations are hard; genu valgum (knock knees) versus genu varum (bowlegs), and some are softer; are the lumbar paraspinals hypertrophied on the right or hypotrophied on the left?

Posture is best understood as being dynamic, adjustable, and responsive to the environment we live and move in. Nevertheless, it is useful to classify static standing posture as a functional baseline. Though individuals may display features of several postural types, there are some classic, common patterns of alignment.

- Note: In acute patients pain compensation patterns will mask underlying posture patterns, so be aware that as the pain of the episode retreats posture may shift dramatically. We suggest posture pictures at the beginning of care, and then following up with new images once someone is out of acute pain.

Posture observations can provide insight to deduce imbalances in the relative contributions of different muscles. However, posture assessment and analysis is as much art as science because in order to balance our body each of us uses a unique combination of our 639 or so muscles. The following information has been garnered from a number of textbooks[7,8,9], as well as clinical experience. The reader is advised to use this information as a starting point to correlate with clinical

CHAPTER FOUR - Posture Assessment Concepts — Posture Pictures

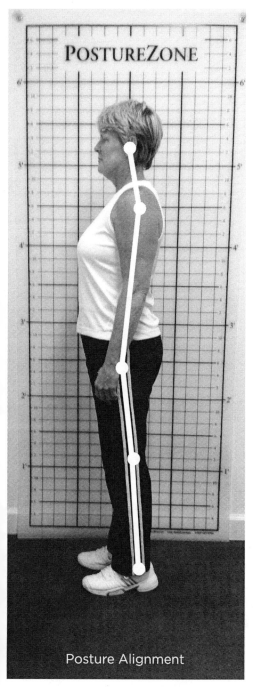

Posture Alignment

findings, testing and observation.

The textbook ideal of good posture has the ears, shoulders, hips, knees and ankles aligned as if a plumb line was running from the:

- Ear (tragus or center)
- Shoulder (bisecting the humerus)
- Hip (ball of femur)
- Knee (just behind center)
- Ankle (center)

The spine should have its normal curves, forward curve in the low back (or lumbar) region (lordosis), backward curve in the mid-back (thoracic) region and forward as the neck (or cervical spine) balances the head on top of the body.

Few people have an ideal body, hence few people have ideal posture. Someone's history, habits and genetics makes their posture unique. In addition, a single posture observation may be the cause, the effect, or a cause of another effect further up, or down, the kinetic chain. Since the body must balance, a posture distortion may be the area of initial injury, or a result of the body compensating to maintain balance. An injury to the knees, ankles or feet may force the body to compensate with hyper-extended knees, which in turn causes knee weakness and wear.

The concept of 4 PostureZones is a useful model based on the simple principles that the body must balance, that it compensates, moves in patterns and adapts. Myriad biomechanical problems can be explained to laypeople using this model, and by looking at posture from the bottom and sequentially assessing the 4 PostureZones.

From bottom to top (feet to head), in clinical posture assessment one should observe the way the:

PostureZone 1:
Lower extremities, which support and balance

PostureZone 2:
Pelvis and low back, which support and balance

PostureZone 3:
Torso and upper extremities, which support and balance

PostureZone 4:
Neck and head.

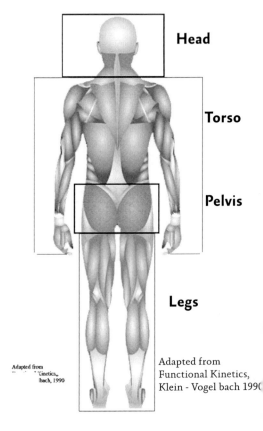

Adapted from Functional Kinetics, Klein - Vogel bach 1990

The 4 PostureZones

Like a stack of children's blocks, we balance from the bottom up. When the blocks are all well-balanced the stack is stable. But when one is out of place, the blocks above are wobbly.

Posture is how you balance your body.

Think about it...if you don't balance, you fall down!

Your posture is quite literally *how* the body balances against gravity. The old nursery rhyme, "the foot bone's connected to the knee bone, the knee bone's connected to the thigh bone," describes the kinetic chain of posture.

To most effectively balance a stack of blocks, you put the second block as squarely as you can on top of the first. Then, you squarely place the third block on the second, because it can only be as stable as the blocks below. Placing a fourth block requires stability of all the blocks that came before it, and so on. As with a set of blocks, the relative alignment and mobility of each posture zone affects how the entire system balances and moves.

> *"Insofar as posture is concerned, the upper body is along for a ride on the pelvic express."* Peter Egoscue[10]

The goal of clinical posture assessment is to first find the tight (or the weak) link in the kinetic chain which is causing something else to compensate, and then focus the patients' or clients' attention to controlled movement and stabilization of that link.

Posture assessment is a trial and error process, and there are often many right answers. However, when it comes to creating the perception of value in the patients mind, as long as follow-up pictures show posture improvement, and especially when there is corresponding clinical improvement, there is a credible perception of value created.

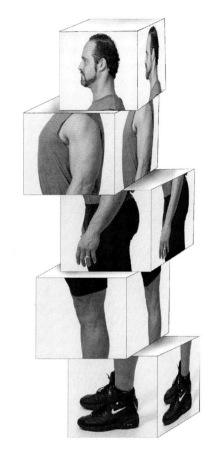

Like a stack of children's blocks, posture must balance from the bottom up

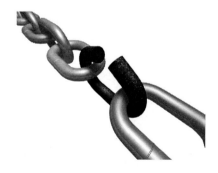

Chain strength is determined by the weak link

CHAPTER FIVE

Posture Assessment

"Show Me Your Best Posture"

When given the instruction "Show me your best posture,"[11] people try and assume what feels like good posture.

Seeing distortions on an image taken when they believe they are standing erect effectively demonstrates the deviation between reality and their perception of good posture. It also serves as a subjectively reproducible starting point for change.

In addition to posed images, pay attention to their resting posture and watch people as they move and stand to catch their "normal" posture.

I suggest first looking at an image with fuzzy vision and asking yourself these questions:

What is not symmetrical from left to right?

1. What sticks out most, and what is off to a lesser degree?
2. Where does there appear to be stress?

Common Clinical Observations

- Right-handed people usually have a low right shoulder and high right hip.
- Left-handed people usually have a low left shoulder and high left hip.
- Side-to-side distortions are common results of adaptations from major and minor injuries and habits such as;
    - carrying a purse on one side,
    - talking on a phone using one shoulder for a cradle,
    - habitually sitting on a fat wallet in a backhip pocket, etc.

Be aware that as you study posture systematically, you'll observe previously overlooked asymmetries and changes.

Scoliosis Note: Spinal curvature along with a high shoulder on one side and a high hip on the other is the classic observation of scoliosis. However, assessment of the different scoliotic patterns is beyond the scope of this book, and we suggest verbally describing an individual's structure as the first step in forming a treatment plan. For scoliosis resources visit:

http://posturezone.com/pages/Resources

Common Observations Well Understood by Patients/Clients

When looking at the functional symmetry, keep in mind the difference between what you as a clinician needs to and is able to observe, and what the patient can see and will find relevant. People understand the structural significance of observations like:

- Centerline alignment
- Uneven Arm-body inter-space
- Hands turned in
- Feet and/or knees asymmetrical

Front View (AP) Posture

AP posture is determined by the spine plus the eight load bearing joints of posture– ankles, knees, hips and shoulders. If your patient or client is not falling down, no matter what, the overall posture MUST be mechanically, physically balanced.

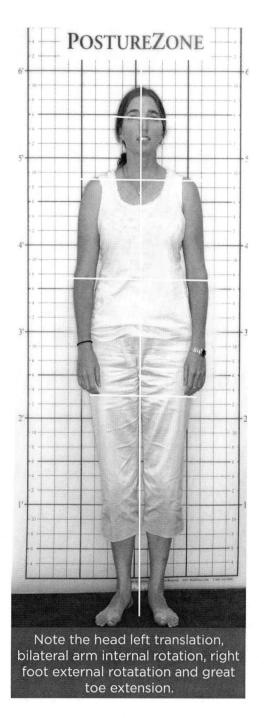

Note the head left translation, bilateral arm internal rotation, right foot external rotatation and great toe extension.

Can you draw a vertical line so it passes evenly between the:

- Eyes
- Chin
- Sternum
- Belly button
- Pubes
- Midway between the knees
- And then evenly between both feet?[12]

Also observe:

- Are the head, shoulders and hips level?
- Are the collar bones symmetric and nearly level?
- Are the arms and hands spaced evenly from the body on both sides?
- Are the knees, ankles and feet angled the same on both sides?
- Can you see the backs of either (or both) hands?

PostureZone Assessment: Front View

The PostureZone model follows a bottom to top logic.

We stand from bottom up and fall from top down.

From bottom to top, note the mechanics of how:

PostureZone 1:
Lower extremities, which support and balance

PostureZone 2:
Pelvis and low back, which support and balance

PostureZone 3:
Torso and upper extremities, which support and balance

PostureZone 4:
Neck and head.
Look at each of the PostureZones from the front, back and side.

When observing posture, for each PostureZone note the appearance of the:

- Center of mass
- Anterior margin
- Posterior margin

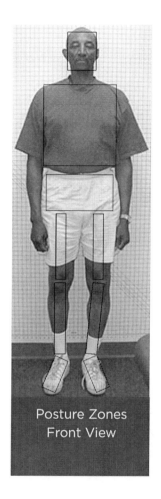

Posture Zones Front View

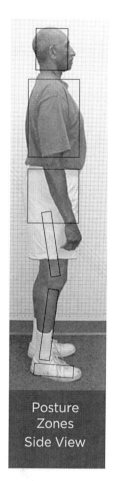

Posture Zones Side View

Posture Pictures
CHAPTER FIVE - Posture Assessment

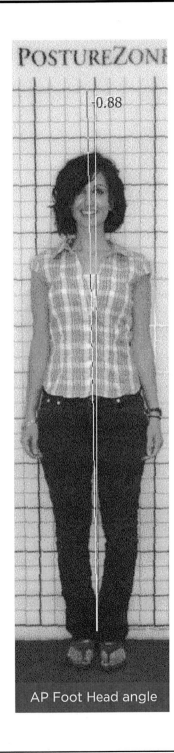

AP Foot Head angle

A technique many professionals find helpful is to compare a line that *should* be vertical and center to *true* vertical and center. The center of mass of each area can then be compared to this reference. Comparison to a theoretic "ideal" plumb line center allows comparison for an individual over a period of time or course of treatment.

So, if we postulate that the center of the head should be over the center of the feet, a comparison of the resulting line with true vertical gives a measurement of the degree of asymmetric posture.

Observations by PostureZone

A basic list of observations follows along with some common muscle patterns of paired tightness/weakness.

BONUS: *See Appendix C for PostureZone Assessment Forms.*

Note: The observations correlate with the findings within the PostureZone Posture Assessment software program

PostureZone 1:
Lower extremity Observations

Are the knees, ankles, and feet angled the same on both sides?

- Does one foot, ankle or knee face differently than its partner? In addition to stressing the feet, ankles and knees, the stress of asymmetric motion travels up the entire kinetic chain, pelvis and spine to head.

- Are the soles of the shoes worn evenly?

    Poor foot posture alters leg biomechanics causing shoes to wear unevenly from one side to the other.

    A common problem affecting many people is feet that roll in, or pronate. A pronated foot has a prominent ankle on the inside, and a sunken one on the outside from the body's weight rolling over the inside edge of the foot.

    Pronators usually benefit from a customized insert for their shoes called an orthotic. Prescription orthotics are manufactured from a cast of your foot, usually taken by a chiropractor, podiatrist or physical therapist. However, many people get a lot of relief from over the counter

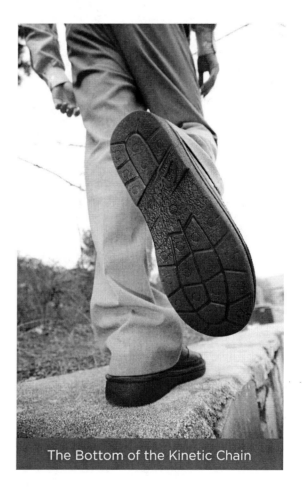

The Bottom of the Kinetic Chain

Posture Pictures   CHAPTER FIVE - Posture Assessment

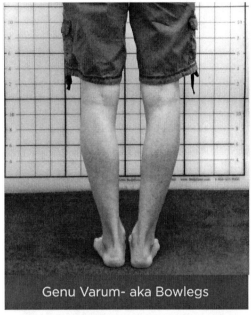

Genu Varum- aka Bowlegs

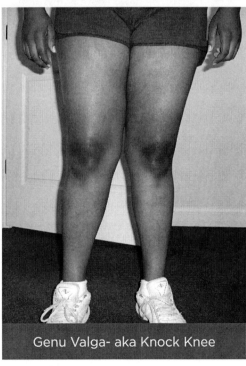

Genu Valga- aka Knock Knee

generic shoe inserts now available online and at specialty shoe care retailers.

Pronators usually wear out their shoes unevenly, with the outside edge of the heel being worn, while the inside edge is like new. This counterintuitive wear pattern results from the way the pronating foot strikes the ground while walking or running. Also, uneven pronation adds further stress as the muscles on the over-pronated side overwork and shorten over time in response to working harder against gravity. When you see an over-pronated foot, the muscles on that side are usually tight.

Shoe wear and orthotics:

- Almost all serious athletes, especially runners, note that their shoes wear more evenly when they use orthotics to balance the biomechanical function of their feet.

- Both knees should face forward, aligning the thigh and calf. Genu varum (bowleg) and Genu valga (knock knee) should be noted.

- Note the relative symmetry of each thigh and calf, as well as any difference in size or rotational alignment.

TABLE 1

Zone 1: Lower Extremity	FRONT VIEW Posture Observations	Possible Associated Tight Muscles	Possible Associated Weak Muscles
Feet	Turn out	Psoas, external hip rotators, sartorius, gluteus maximus	TFL, gluteus minimus
	Pronate	Peroneus	Tibialis anterior, tibialis posterior
	Supination	Tibialis anterior, tibialis posterior	Peroneals
	Clench/ hammer toes	Plantar fascia	Anterior tibialis
Knees	Hyper-extension	Hamstrings, gastrocnemius	Lower quadriceps, popliteus
	External Knee rotation	TFL, gluteus medius	Gluteus maximus, sartorius, tibialis anterior
	Genu Vara/ bowlegs	Gluteus medius, tensor fascia lata	Adductors, gluteus medius
	Genu Valga/ knock knees	Adductors, gluteus medius	Gluteus medius, tensor fascia lata
Thighs	IT band groove	Ilio-tibial band/ TFL	Thigh adductors

PostureZone 2: Pelvis

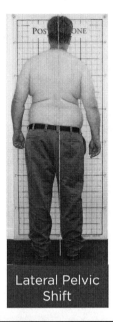

Lateral Pelvic Shift

Is the pelvis shifted to one side?

- Indicates tightness or imbalance of the thigh muscles (TFL/ITB) or weakness of the deep hip muscles (gluteus medius).
- Note: A background posture grid helps visualize laterality even if an image is not perfectly aligned.

TABLE 2

Zone 2: Pelvis	FRONT VIEW Posture Observations	Possible Associated Tight Muscles	Possible Associated Weak Muscles
	Umbilicus deviation (likely associated with pelvic distortion) (possibly indicative of visceral disorder)	Abdominals (usually secondary to other pelvic distortions)	Contralateral abdominals
	Pelvic drop / high on one side	Quadratus lumborum, psoas	Contralateral quadratus lumborum, psoas
	Pelvic posterior/ backwards rotation	Abdominus oblique, psoas, TFL, sartorius	Contralateral abdominus oblique, psoas, TFL, sartorius

PostureZone 3: Torso

Are the arms and hands spaced evenly from the body on both sides?

- If one arm is touching the body and one is not, or if the arms are not equally spaced from the body, then either the shoulders are not over the pelvis (as discussed above), or the shoulders are not sitting on the chest symmetrically.

- Uneven carriage of the shoulders can result from always sleeping on the same side or repetitive work habits. The school bus driver who always uses one arm to push the handle to open a door, the carpenter who always hammers with his right hand, and the secretary who always reaches the same awkward way to use her mouse in a poorly designed workstation are all training their body to have weak posture.

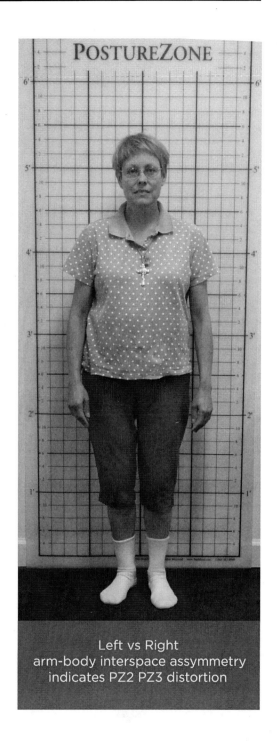

Left vs Right
arm-body interspace assymmetry indicates PZ2 PZ3 distortion

Can you see the backs of either (or both) hands?

- When standing straight, from the front you should only see the thumb side of the hands, with back of the hands and the pinky finger mostly hidden behind the hand. If you can see the backs of the hands, it usually means the shoulders are rounded forward (internally rotated). This is a very common observation, especially when there is a Forward Head Posture observed from the side view.

TABLE 3

Zone 3: Torso	FRONT VIEW Posture Observations	Possible Associated Tight Muscles	Possible Associated Weak Muscles
Chest	Breathing pattern Chest or chest assist	Scalenes, levator scap, serratus posterior superior	Diaphragm, transverse abdominals, serratus posterior inferior
	Back Rounded/ flat	Pectorals	Rhomboids, mid/ lower trap
Shoulders	Assymmetric clavicular grooves	Scalene assymmetry	Scalene assymmetry
Arms	Arms forward of body	Upper Trap, levator scap	mid and lower trap
	Arms rolled in/ tight arm-body space	Pectorals, lats, teres major, subscapularis	Teres minor, infraspinatus

PostureZone 4:

Head: Is the head level and balanced above the shoulders?

- Forward head posture (FHP) is an epidemic in our society, and is arguably the most common and problematic posture adaptation.
- On Front and Back view images, when someone appears to be "looking up" or in an extension adaptation, they are demonstrating a classic Forward head posture observation. When asked to show you their "best posture", they perceive their head is forward of the body and so attempt to "correct", although they are actually pulling the head backwards into extension

Note: Neck retractions are an exercise to counter this adaptation in the StrongPosture™ and other posture exercise protocols.[13]

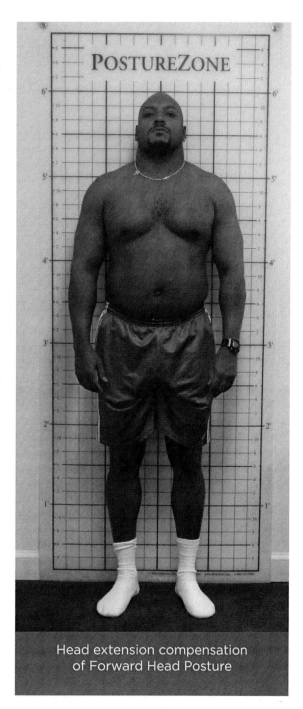

Head extension compensation of Forward Head Posture

TABLE 4

Zone 4: Head	FRONT VIEW Posture Observations	Possible Associated Tight Muscles	Possible Associated Weak Muscles
	Lateral tilt &/or rotation	SCM, upper trapezius, levator scap	Contralateral SCM, upper trapezius, levator scap
	TMJ distortion	Pterygoid muscles, masseters	Contralateral pterygoid muscles, masseters
Neck	SCM hypertrophy	SCM	Deep neck flexors
	Neck short on a side	Upper trap, levator scap, levator	Contralateral upper trap, levator, ipsilateral mid/lower trap
	Forward head posture	Sub occipitals, SCM, pectorals, upper traps	Deep neck flexors, mid-lower traps, rhomboids

Back (Posterior) View Observations

As in the front view, the body should appear equal from left to right. When a body is well aligned, a vertical line should be centered. Ideally, you should be able to draw a vertical line through:

- Center of the skull (Occipital protuberance)
- With alignment thru the neck
- Vertebral prominens (C7/T1 spinous process, the bump at the base of the neck) with alignment of the middle back
- Evenly between both shoulder blades
- Evenly between both hips and between the gluteal folds
- Between both knees
- Evenly between the feet

In balanced posture, a line drawn between the following structures should be parallel:

- Tips of the mastoid processes
- Top of the shoulders/acromion processes
- Scapula
- Lower margins of the 12th ribs
- Top of iliac crests/ Posterior superior iliac spines

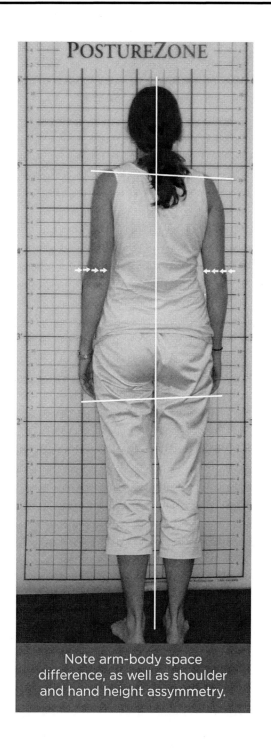

Note arm-body space difference, as well as shoulder and hand height assymmetry.

- Ischial tuberosities
- Back of the knees

The legs should be symmetrical with the backs of the knees equal. Ankles and feet should be equally aligned with respect to pronation/supination and toe in/toe out.

Arm-body interspace should be equal on both sides with arms hanging symmetrically from the torso, with an equal and small amount of the palms visible.

> Demonstrating the correlation between slumping postures and the degree of internal arm rotation can effectively show the biomechanics and create an understanding of the consequences of adaptive posture.

Note: Most people have a slight postural asymmetry due to left or right hand dominance. Right-handed people tend towards a high right hip, a low right shoulder and a slight right convex thoracic curve. Left-handed individuals tend to have a high left hip, a low left shoulder and a slight left convex thoracic curve.

TABLE 5

Zone 4: Head	BACK VIEW Posture Observations By Zone	Possible Associated Tight Muscles	Possible Associated Weak Muscles
Neck	Lateral tilt &/or rotation	SCM, upper trapezius, levator scap	Contralateral SCM, upper trapezius, levator scap
	SCM hypertrophy R___ L___	SCM	Deep neck flexors
	Short neck	Upper trap, levator scap, levator	Contralateral upper trap, levator, ipsilateral mid/lower trap
	Forward head posture	Sub occipitals, SCM, pectorals, upper traps	Deep neck flexors, mid-lower traps, rhomboids
	Forward head posture	Sub occipitals, SCM, pectorals, upper traps	Deep neck flexors, mid-lower traps, rhomboids
Zone 3: Torso	**Upper back rounded/ marked kyphosis (hunchback)**	**Pectorals, upper traps, rectus abdominais**	**Mid and lower trap, rhomboids**
Upper Extremity	Upper back flattened	Lumbar erector spinae, hamstrings,	Rhomboids, mid/lower trap

Shoulders	Scapula Winging	Serratus anterior, pectorals, ant. deltoid	Middle traps, rhomboids
	Scapula external rotation	Serratus anterior, upper traps	Mid and lower trap, rhomboid
Arms	Arms forward	Upper trap, levator scap, pectoralis	Mid and lower trap
	Rolled in/ tight arm-body space	Pectorals, lats, teres major, subscapularis	Teres minor, infraspinatus
Zone 2: Pelvis	**Mid-back and low back spinal muscles**	**Paraspinal and deep spinal MM, QL, hip flexors**	**Contralateral back muscles, abdominals**
	Pelvic drop, (aka. high on one side)	Quadratus lumborum, psoas	Contralateral quadratus lumborum, psoas
	Pelvic rotation posterior, (backwards)	Abdominus oblique, psoas, TFL, sartorius	Contralateral abdominus oblique, psoas, TFL, sartorius
	Scapula external rotation	Serratus anterior, upper traps	Mid and lower trap, rhomboid
Zone 1: Lower Extremity	**IT Band Groove**	**TFL**	**Adductors**
Knees	Hyper-extension	Hamstrings, gastrocnemius	Lower quadriceps. Popliteus
	External Knee rotation	TFL, gluteus medius	Gluteus maximus, sartorius, tibialis anterior

Feet	Genu valga/ bowlegs	Gluteus medius, tensor fascia lata	Adductors, gluteus medius
	Genu vara/ knock knees	Adductors, gluteus medius	Gluteus medius, tensor fascia lata
	Turn out	Psoas, external hip rotators, sartorius, gluteus maximus	TFL, gluteus minimus
	Pronate	Peroneal	Tibialis anterior, tibialis posterior
	Supination	Tibialis anteriot tibialis posterior	Peroneals
	Clench/ hammer toes	Plantar fascia	Anterior tibialis

Posture Pictures CHAPTER FIVE - Posture Assessment

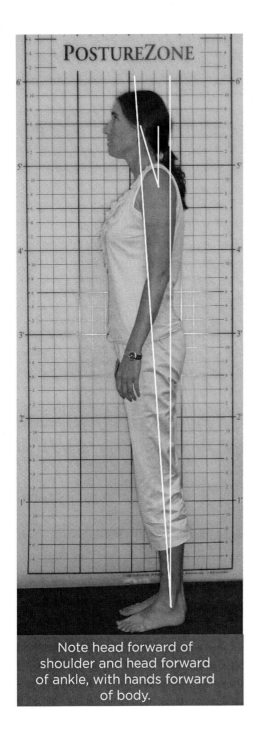

Note head forward of shoulder and head forward of ankle, with hands forward of body.

Side (lateral) View Posture Observations

There are three concepts of lateral posture evaluations:

1. How is the body shifting its weight in order to balance?
2. How does the resulting compensation and adaptation affect the front contour of the body?
3. How does the resulting compensation and adaptation affect the back contour of the body?

Balance Observations

- Is the center of mass (CoM) of the head level and balanced above the shoulders?
- Are the shoulders level and directly above the hips?
- Are the arms resting at the side, with the back of the hand fully visible?
- Is the chest elevated or depressed?
- Are the hips level, or is the pelvis tilted forwards or backwards?
- Are the hips, knees and feet aligned?

Front (Anterior) body contour observations:

- Is the head forward of the chest?
- Is the chest depressed?
- Is the belly large and protruding?
- Is the pelvis pushed forward?

Back (Posterior) body contour observations:

- Is the head forward of the chest?
- Are the shoulders rounded?
- Do one or both of the shoulder blades "wing out"?
- Does the low back curve forward (swayback) or flatten (flat back)?
- Are the buttocks rounded or flat, or tilted forward or back?

Common Observations Well Understood by Patients/Clients

- Earlobe should be in line with the shoulder
- Shoulder should be in line with the hip
- Ear should be in line with the ankle

Posture Pictures | CHAPTER FIVE - Posture Assessment

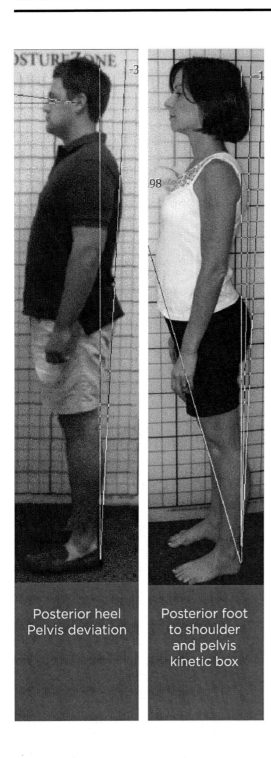

Posterior heel
Pelvis deviation

Posterior foot
to shoulder
and pelvis
kinetic box

PostureZone Assessment: Side View

Remember: the body is always balancing. When looking at a body from the side, the question to ask is, "How?"

Noting what is moved forward and what is moved back in order to balance can give tremendous insight into someone's habits and past injuries, as well as their current problems and complaints.

Look at the side-view picture, from the bottom up, and note in each PostureZone:

- Center of mass
- Anterior margin
- Posterior margin

A technique many professionals find helpful is to compare with true vertical a line from the back of the heel to the:

- Pelvis
- Torso / Shoulders
- Head

Similarly, the center of mass of each area can be compared to the anterior ankle (the theoretic "ideal" plumb line center). Within an individual over a period of time, or course of treatment, comparing the angle between true vertical and the angle created by the line running between the ankle and the:

- Center of Hip
- Center of Torso / Shoulder
- Center of Ear

Observe the following and consider how:

- PostureZone 4: Head and neck, balances on
- PostureZone 3: Torso and upper extremity, which balance on
- PostureZone 2: Low back and pelvis, which balances on
- PostureZone 1: Lower extremities

For each PostureZone common findings are noted.

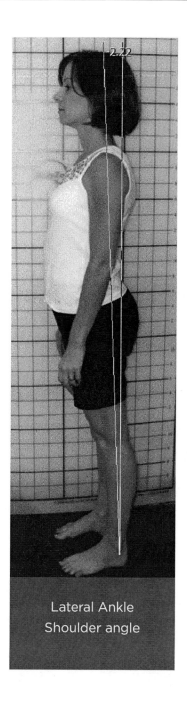

Lateral Ankle Shoulder angle

PostureZone 1:

Lower extremity: Are the hips, knees, and feet aligned?

- Are the hips directly above knees, and the knees above, or just slightly forward, of the ankles?
- In neutral posture, the thighs and calves should be roughly vertical.

TABLE 6

Zone 1: Lower Extremity	Side View PostureZone Observation	Possible Associated Tight Muscles	Possible Associated Weak Muscles
Knees	Knees hyper-extended	Hamstrings, gastrocnemius	Popliteus, quadriceps

PostureZone 2:

Pelvis: Are the hips level, or is the pelvis tilted forward, or backward? Does the belly protrude?

- There is dramatic postural difference between how a person stands when the pelvis is level, and when they are arching back because the pelvis is tilting forward. Especially when someone is overweight, the pelvis tilts forward (anterior tilt).

- Not all people with protruding abdomens are overweight. Many people in good shape have a protruding abdomen, and roll their pelvis forward. Fit or fat, the body has to balance.

- Forward tilts also occur from chronic sitting postures. Folding the body in a sitting position shortens the muscles in front of the hips (the flexors) and lengthens the muscles behind the hips (the extensors).

- If someone has tight hip flexors, a rolled-in chest, or other common posture distortions, they must compensate and adapt. A protruding abdomen pulls the pelvis forward, rolling the pelvis into a forward tilt. When the pelvis rolls forward, the shoulders and torso shift back to keep you from falling onto your face. The head then juts forward to compensate and balance. (Visualize again a wobbly stack of children's building blocks)

According to mass media imagery, a flat stomach is the holy grail of fitness. Late night television ads promise patients and clients that they too can have "six-pack, washboard abs" by purchasing an ab-roller, belly blaster, six-pack cutter, or other gimmicky exercise contraption, lotion, or potion. And, each year there are a host of new products promising to make the process easier still, if not effortless. So why do many people who are in good shape still work unsuccessfully to have a flat stomach? The answer frequently is in their posture.

Many people who complain of "tired backs" or "weak abs" have reported dramatic relief after learning to balance with stronger posture. Of course, this means you have to become conscious of your posture, which is one very good reason to take a side view posture picture during your patient's / client's assessment.

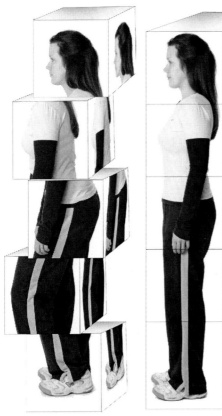

Weak unbalanced posture

Strong balanced posture

TABLE 7

Zone 2: Pelvis	Side View PostureZone Observation	Possible Associated Tight Muscles	Possible Associated Weak Muscles
	Backward weight balance	Tibialis anterior psoas, rectus abdominis	Gluteus maximus, thoracic erector spinae
	Forward weight balance	Gluteus maximus, thoracic erector spinae	Tibialis anterior psoas, rectus abdominis
	Forward pelvic tilt	Psoas , rectus femoris	gluteus medius, minimus, abdominals (especially TrA)
Low Back	Flattened	Middle trapezius. rectus abdominis	Lumbar erectors, psoas, hip flexors
	Increased lordotic arch	Lumbar erectors, psoas, hip flexors	Middle trapezius, rectus abdominis
Abdomen	Protruding	Erector spinae	Abdominals
	Supination	Tibialis anteriot tibialis posterior	Peroneals
	Clench/ hammer toes	Plantar fascia	Anterior tibialis

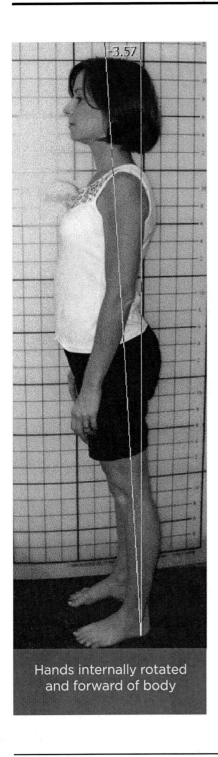

Hands internally rotated and forward of body

PostureZone 3:

Torso: Are the shoulders level and even with the hips?

- Your posture is how you balance your body, so if your shoulders are not over your hips, you are working harder than you should to hold yourself up.

- Is the chest elevated or depressed?

- Is the arm resting at the side, with the back of the hand visible? Or, is the pinky side of the hand hiding the thumb, indicating internal rotation of the shoulder?

Forward, rolled-in shoulders frequently accompany Forward Head Posture because in our society people keep their hands close together to compute, text, drive and do many other modern tasks.

When the arms are in front of the body, the shoulders are rolled forward and the chest depresses (typical texting posture). As the hands and eyes follow the shoulders forward into the classic rounded shoulder forward head posture (Upper Cross Syndrome), the chest is compressed. Ultimately, taking a deep breath can become difficult due to limited chest expansion.

TABLE 8

Zone 3: Torso	Side View PostureZone Observation	Possible Associated Tight Muscles	Possible Associated Weak Muscles
Chest	Chest depressed	Pectorals	Rhomboids, mid/lower trap
	Back flat	Pectorals, traps	Latissimus dorsi, rhomboid
Upper Extremity Shoulders	Shoulders rolled in	Pectorals, serratus anterior	Middle and lower trapezius, latissimus dorsi
Arms	Shoulders forward	Upper trap, levator scap	Mid and lower trap
	Shoulders rolled in/ tight arm-body space	Pectorals, lats, teres major, subscapularis	Teres minor, infraspinatus
Abdomen	Protruding	Erector spinae	Abdominals
	Supination	Tibialis anteriot tibialis posterior	Peroneals
	Clench/ hammer toes	Plantar fascia	Anterior tibialis

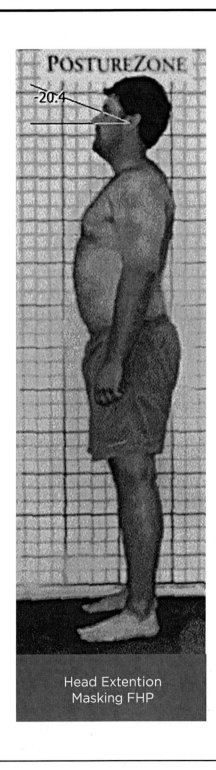

Head Extention Masking FHP

PostureZone 4:

Head: Is the head level and balanced above the shoulders?.

- Is the head level or in extension?
- Is the hard palate level with the floor?
- Are the eyes looking at a point straight ahead?

People will often mask their forward head posture with head extension

Forward head posture causes chronic problems like neck pain, headaches, and arm pain and contributes to conditions ranging from osteoarthritis in the neck to carpal tunnel syndrome.

For every inch that the head moves forward of the torso, the weight of the head carried by the lower neck and upper back doubles, according to some experts. The computer worker, the student, the commuter, the couch potato slumping in his recliner, have all trained their bodies to balance despite this increased biomechanical stress and strain.

The predictable result is adaptive overwork and tightness of some neck, upper back, and shoulder muscles; atrophy of other muscles, and over time, premature breakdown and degeneration of the spine and other joints.

TABLE 9

Zone 4: Head	Side View PostureZone Observation	Possible Associated Tight Muscles	Possible Associated Weak Muscles
Neck	Forward head posture/ extension adaptation (usually associated with loss of cervical curve)	Sub occipitals, SCM, pectorals, upper traps	Deep neck flexors, mid-lower traps, rhomboids, serratus anterior

CHAPTER SIX

Communicating Posture Findings

In Office Screening / Report of Findings

When a patient's first visit includes a posture picture, it is an integral part of the report process. Have a staff person give the patient their posture picture to look at while they are waiting. People find pictures of themselves intensely interesting, especially lateral views showing their true posture... remember, they *thought* they were standing straight.

Give the patient a copy of their posture picture, and put another one in their file for your documentation, and follow up. In addition, keep the electronic copy for evaluating progress, comparison on re-exam and for annual posture pictures.

Simply taking a posture picture sharpens someone's posture awareness, which then grows as they progress... from pain relief to rehab, along a performance enhancement program, or learning to integrate posture exercise for anti-aging benefits.

Posture aware patients and clients often report they're standing taller with postural therapy. In a clinical setting, creating posture awareness during AcuteCare is key to transitioning patients to WellnessCare, and is pivotal in their decision to adopt a daily life habit of posture exercises.

Re-exam and Annual Posture Pictures

Take follow up posture pictures periodically, especially when shifting phase of care. In addition, a recall/reactivation effort with an offer of a no-charge annual posture picture provides the opportunity to compare this year's posture picture with previous pictures.

Looking at posture can give a tremendous amount of information about how a body is working. Some studies show weak reproducibility in posture image findings due to the difficulty in finding a change significantly larger than baseline repositioning errors.[14] In my opinion, lateral posture views using hard tissue references showed the best reproducibility of findings and are the most valuable posture view.

Note forward hand and torso

After 2 weeks of posture therapy symptoms and photo are improved

CHAPTER SIX - Communicating Posture Findings — Posture Pictures

In addition to reproducibility, the overlapping causes and effects of a lifetime's habits and injuries make assessment an art as well as a science. In practice, posture pictures are not the only thing we hang our metaphorical hat on. Physical exam and testing, x-ray and other evaluation procedures and tests are all part of building a clinical picture. If you teach postural exercise, look carefully at a person's ability to effectively perform exercises with control and symmetry.

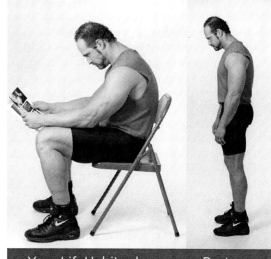
Your LifeHabits shape your Posture

As the patient or client becomes more posture conscious they begin to kinesthetically feel a difference in how they are performing an exercise, and that ability improves with postural therapies that unlock tight links in their kinetic chain.

Coupled with improved one leg balance function, on re-exam the dialogue is not merely "the posture picture says you are better", but rather "We can both see, and you can feel that your posture is stronger and your balance and motion control are improved."

For more information on communicating posture, balance and motion concepts to clients and patients review the Five Posture Principles in Appendix B.

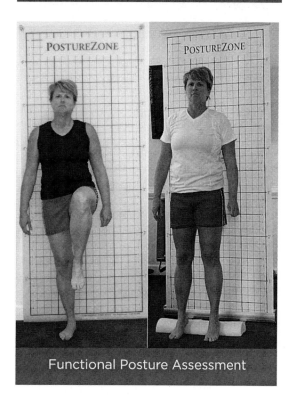
Functional Posture Assessment

Public Posture Screenings

People are interested in their posture, so posture pictures are a popular tool at health fairs, school scoliosis screens, gyms, senior centers and other venues. At public events appearance is vital to building trust and credibility. This is the time to invest in professional materials. Tacky signage and outdated brochures should be discarded in favor of new signs or banners and crisp, educational information.

Good planning requires an Intake Form. This form should include a very short blurb marketing your practice, gather basic contact information for follow-up, and a release allowing you to take the image and discuss your findings while releasing you from any liability. *(Disclaimer: It is your sole responsibility to contact legal counsel to check the necessity, wording, and requirements for your profession and state prior to setting up or using any release form.)* It's a great idea to include an option to 'sign up now' for your informative newsletter by simply checking a box.

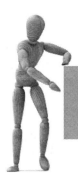

BONUS: See Appendix D for Posture Assessment Intake Forms

If you plan to run the reports after the event, we strongly recommend having a system, such as using the back of the intake form to indicate information to help you easily identify the subject when processing the posture assessments. (Note clothing, hair color, or other easily identifiable information.) Be sure any description you put in writing is positive and professional.

You'll take the posture assessment photo at the event, but it's up to you whether to give the person a take home report at the venue, email it to them after the event, or make an in-office appointment to discuss the results of their analysis. Whatever you choose, the goal is to use the opportunity to create posture consciousness, and explore the biomechanical connections between any symptoms they are suffering and their posture adaptations.

- The teacher with a tight middle back more than likely has a marked forward head posture, causing the middle back muscles to be overworked, straining to support the neck.

- The runner with the low back pain likely has some asymmetry of the lower extremity, creating low back stress from training the body to balance on unevenly developed legs.

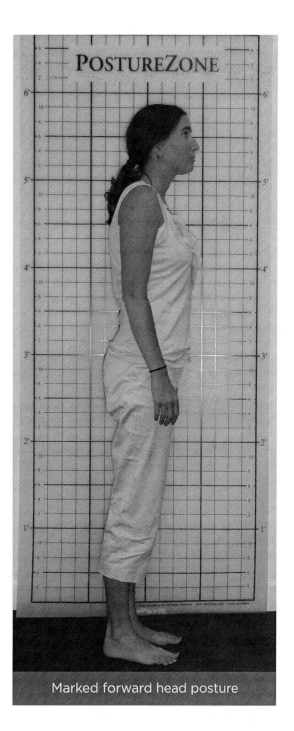

Marked forward head posture

- The 60 year old woman with "normal" low back pain with bilaterally short psoas from a chronic forward flexion posture may be shocked to see how far forward she is flexing, and knows her now hunched-over mother once looked as she does now.

When you talk to people about posture they often shift about and pull their shoulders back to "stand straight". When they do, some may feel tightness in the shoulders and others may feel tightness in the legs, low back or wherever the tight link is in their body. The challenge is pointing out and connecting this tight link with their symptoms.

People want to learn...so at an event your goal is to teach them, and to communicate the benefits linking your services with their posture improvement.

CHAPTER SEVEN

Setting Up Posture Screenings

Marketing Posture Assessments Outside the Office

Screenings are engaging and provide participants with valuable information about their posture and motion patterns. A multitude of businesses and groups may be interested in hosting your posture screening at their facility, meeting or event.

It's important to identify the cross-marketing opportunities between your services and the prospective host's services or products *before* you call or meet to discuss your ideas. Tailor your proposal to the prospective host to highlight the benefits to their business. What is the value to the host business or group, and the appeal for their clientele, employees or members?

- Will you focus your communications at the sporting goods store to correlate your findings and services with their in-store products?
- Could the Country Club advertise that they are "sponsoring the posture screening" as a special service to improve their members golf swing?

There's real value in the posture assessment you'll provide. Emphasize how your services complement and mesh with *(not compete with)* the prospective host's services or products. Remember, this should be the beginning of a win-win relationship, you want people to speak well of you after you leave *(referrals)* and you want to be invited back *(more referrals)*.

Here is a chart to illustrate just a few ways a posture assessment screening would benefit the customers, employees, patients or members of a variety of businesses, practitioners and groups. Use this information to brainstorm how your services might synergize with and complement their services.

Prospective Posture Screening Venue	How Posture Fits Their Audience
Business	
• Fitness clubs and gyms	Function, avoid injury, interactive event
• Sporting Goods stores	Function, enhanced sports performance, properly using store products and equipment
• Golf and tennis specialty stores	Strength, performance, improved game
• Health Food Store	Interactive event, health conscious, wellness

• Golf Course, Driving range, Pro Shop	Improved swing and consistency, range of motion, added benefit for members
• Instructor Studio, Yoga, Pilates, etc.	Balance, flexibility, body awareness
• Personal/Athletic Trainer	Strong foundation, symmetry, balance
• Dance Instruction	Poise, grace, flexibility, symmetry, balance, injury preven
• Vocal Coach	Effects on breathing, stage presence
• Modeling School	Symmetry, poise and aesthetics (beauty)
• Large corporations	Computing forward-folded posture creates pain, impacting productivity, avoiding repetitive stress injury.
Health	
• Chiropractic	Alignment, muscle imbalance, pain relief, function, wellness, range of motion
• MD, DO	Function, wellness, activity prescription
• Podiatry	Balance, uneven wear, gait, foundation
• Dental	TMJ, Oro-myologic postural asymmetry, breathing

• Physical / Physio Therapy	Symmetry of motion, flexibility, functional imbalance
• Massage Therapist, Rolfer	Muscle imbalance, tightness, flexibility
• Alexander Technique, Feldenkrais	Visualize functional effects of harmful habits
• Hospitals	Posture awareness in workplace, pain/injury avoidance, productivity
• Senior Living Facility, activity director	Participation, increased activity, balance, longevity, breathing capacity, interactive event
Events	
• Health fairs, community or hospital	Health, wellness, interactive, all age groups
• Community festivals	Posture assessments are interactive, valuable take-home info, health/family related
Groups	
• Rotary, Kiwanis	Anti-aging, pain relief, interactive meeting activity
• Moms	Lifting, pain relief, post-pregnancy posture
• Church meeting groups	Interactive, educational, health/family related
• Senior Centers	Balance, active aging, engaging event

• Community Centers, YMCA	Interactive activity, educational, fitness related
• Business (networking, real estate, etc)	Computing ergonomics, neck strain, interactive break-out activity
Athletic Groups	
• Tennis (ALTA, etc)	Strength, precision, consistency, pain relief
• Runners	Endurance, function, strain, uneven joint wear, pain relief
• Rowers, Cyclists	Performance, effects of sitting posture
Schools, Public and Private	
• Annual Screenings	Scoliosis screenings, posture awareness
• Backpack awareness	Posture awareness, injury avoidance
• Computing/Gaming awareness	Effects of forward-folded posture, awareness, pain relief, flexibility
• Athletic teams	Enhanced performance, avoid injury, strength
• Cheerleaders	Performance, balance, injury avoidance, poise
• Teachers	Standing/sitting posture, pain relief, ergonomics, productivity

Resources for Locating Prospective Venues

Business & Health:

The print business telephone directory is a good place to start. Look up every category suggested above and start making your list of prospective contacts.

Use an internet map service to locate more businesses in your vicinity. Two of the best are *maps.google.com* and *www.mapquest.com*.

Contact the Chamber of Commerce to get a list of new businesses in the area.

Hospitals:

Many hospitals offer periodic health screenings, fairs and events. Once you've identified all of the hospitals in your area, visit their websites for a listing of coming events offered to the general public.

Events:

Check out your city government website to view the event calendar for upcoming community festivals and fairs at the town or city center. While online, be on the lookout for a link to the parks and recreation department, they usually have a separate website and listings for activities they organize.

www.craigslist.com is a popular website with a limited community section that advertises events, classes, activities and groups.

www.eventful.com is a website dedicated to promoting events of all types, they have sections for both health and community.

www.zvents.com offers listings for education & classes, community, outdoor & fitness, and festivals.

Local newspaper, television and radio stations host websites with current information of popular happenings around town.

Groups:

www.meetup.com is an excellent resource for finding and connecting with private social groups in your area. The website is designed to help people with like interests form groups and plan activities together.

- A quick zip code search on meetup.com will return dozens *(sometimes hundreds)* of results describing groups, interests, meeting times and number of active members.

- You'll find everything from stay-at-home moms, to runners, cyclists and hikers, to vegetarians and business strategy groups. Read the description of each group and determine why a posture screening would benefit the members.

Schools:

You'll find a complete listing of public, private and charter schools on your state government website. (find your state website using search term: *your state .gov*)

After the Screening

Since groups often set up events months in advance, an annual Posture Screening & Marketing Calendar is a necessity for the successful posture practice.

At the end of an event, remember to thank the host venue…and ask to be contacted when they start planning next year's schedule. Make a note on your calender to follow up.

Especially when you return to an event year after year, posture screenings are a great way to build community relationships and position yourself as the local Posture Expert.

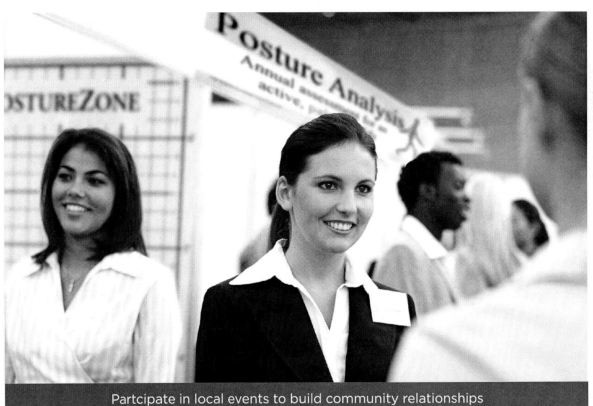
Partcipate in local events to build community relationships

APPENDICES

Appendix A   Marketing Flyers
Appendix B   The Five Posture Principles
Appendix C   Posture Assessment Forms
Appendix D   Patient/Client Intake Form

Appendix A: Why Posture is Important - Marketing Flyer
Download customizable version at:
www.posturezone.com/pages/book

Posture Analysis

Annual assessment for an active, pain-free life

IDENTIFY THE CAUSE

POOR POSTURE
- Back Pain
- Neck Pain
- Stiff Joints
- Headache
- Arthritis

LET'S TALK ABOUT THE SOLUTION

STRONG POSTURE™
- Balance
- Alignment
- Motion

Why Posture Is Important

Everyone knows posture is important for effective relief of body and muscle aches, yet many people are surprised to learn strengthening posture can improve sports performance, and even help people age well.

Your posture is HOW you balance your body. In other words, how the HEAD balances on the TORSO which balances on the PELVIS which balances on the LEGS.

Like a stack of children's blocks, the alignment and mobility of each of The 4 PostureZones affects how the entire body balances and moves.

Poor posture alignment and uneven motion contribute to the mechanical stress on the body. Problems from chronic muscle and joint aches and pains from the feet to the neck can result in premature joint breakdown (i.e. osteoarthritis).

Strengthening posture with professional care and StrongPosture- exercise reduces bio-mechanical posture stress to help conditions from back pain and sciatica to tension headaches, while also improving athletic performance and promoting pain-free activity.

BodyZone Training Center
3000 Old Alabama Rd
Suite 119-352
Alpharetta GA 30022
www.bodyzone.com
mail@bodyzone.com

©2011 BodyZone.com All Rights Reserved 770-922-0700

Appendix A: Posture Analysis Marketing
Download customizable version at:
www.posturezone.com/pages/book

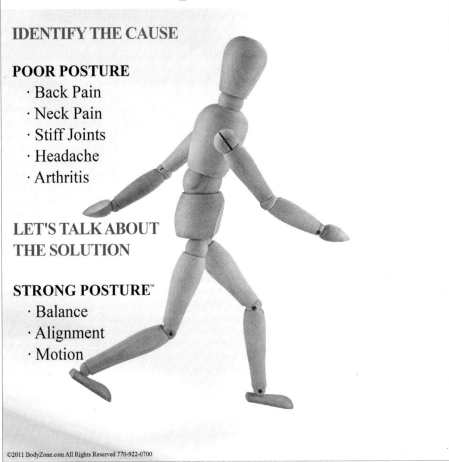

Appendix A: Posture Analysis Marketing Flyer
Download full size color copy at:
www.posturezone.com/pages/book

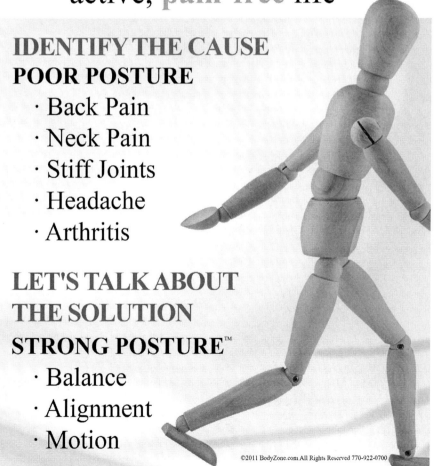

Appendix A: It All Begins with an Assessment - Marketing Flyer
Download full size color copy at:
www.posturezone.com/pages/book

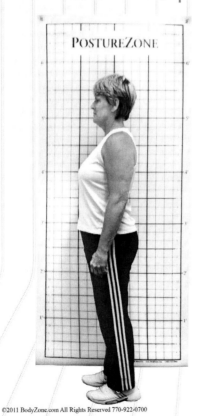

Appendix A: Posture Analysis Flyer - For Your Event or Offer
Download customizable version at:
www.posturezone.com/pages/book

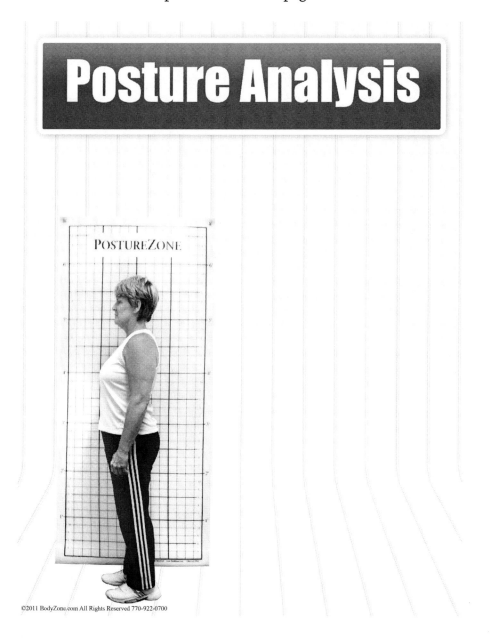

Appendix B

The Principles Of Posture & Body Motion

THE 1ST POSTURE PRINCIPLE, MOTION

THE HUMAN BODY IS DESIGNED TO MOVE

The body's motion is controlled by the neuro-musculo-skeletal system (NMS system). The NMS, also known as the motion system, is composed of:

- Bones: to hold the body up
- Ligaments: to hold the bones together at the joints
- Tendons: to hold the muscles to the bone
- Cartilage, discs, and synovial fluid: to protect and lubricate the joints
- Muscles: to move the bones
- Fascia: (the stuff that holds it all together)
- The brain and nervous system: to tell the muscles what to do

Another way of looking at the motion system is to group the different tissues together by their function, or what they do. When arranged by function, the tissues of the Motion system can be logically grouped into 3 categories, or subsystems.

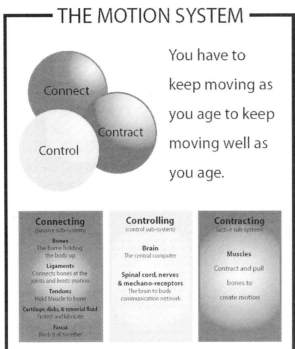

The Three Motion System Subsystems are:

- The Contracting (technically known as the Active) Subsystem
  Consists of the muscles, which create motion.
- The Connecting (technically known as the Passive) Subsystem
  This includes the skeleton, ligaments, tendons, Fascla, and other connective tissue holding the body together.
- The Control Subsystem
  Consists of the brain, spinal cord, nerves & mechanoreceptors, which control motion.

All the components of the motion system must work together, with integrated function, for normal, healthy motion. The Motion system works as a single system. If you have strong muscles (or Contracting system) you are not fit and healthy unless there is an equally strong Connecting and Control subsystems. The weightlifter with strong biceps, but a bad elbow, is not going to lift one ounce more weight than his elbow allows.

When you keep your body moving, joints work fully and freely, muscles stay limber, and you stay active as you age. Balanced and Full Motion allows joints and muscles to move smoothly, in their full normal range.

You must keep moving well as you age to keep moving well as you age.

Problems with motion affect the contracting, connecting and control subsystems. To effectively help a motion problem, intelligent solutions must address the mechanical as well as the neurological.

Chiropractic adjustments unlock, restore and maintain joint motion. By mobilizing joints (frequently in the spine, but other joints too) the chiropractor reduces spinal joint misalignment and other posture and motion distortions. In fact, freeing a compressed nerve or restoring motion can affect other parts of the body via the control subsystem.

Massage Therapy lengthens tight muscles and breaks up ligamentous and fascial adhesions. Massage techniques such as deep tissue, neuromuscular therapy, cross-fiber technique, ART™, Graston™, Rolfing and trigger point are effective at opening restrictions of the contracting subsystem. Other benefits can be pain relief, which affects the control subsystem, improved circulation, and general stress reduction.

Posture exercise as a daily LifeHabit trains the body to keep moving with conscious, full range motion.

THE 2ND POSTURE PRINCIPLE, BALANCE

POSTURE IS HOW YOU BALANCE YOUR BODY

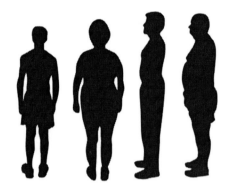

If you don't balance, you fall down. Your posture, and your body motion, may not be symmetrical, but, if you are not falling down, it must be balanced. You may be working hard to stand up, but ultimately your posture is balancing your body. Stable and Strong Posture promotes balanced motion.

THE 3RD POSTURE PRINCIPLE, PATTERNS

THE PATTERN OF A BODY'S CHAIN OF MOTION FOLLOWS THE PATH OF LEAST RESISTANCE

A chain is no stronger than its weakest link, and life is after all a chain. William James (1842-1910) The body moves in a chain of motion, also known as a kinetic chain.

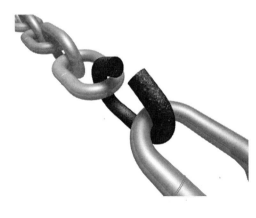

Bones move when connecting muscles contract, pulling one bone toward another. Motion occurs when the force of contraction is greater than the resistance. When the body moves in space, posture must shift in order to maintain balance, requiring changed muscle activity. This shifting is usually unconscious. Muscles become strong when used or trained for a specific activity, but we don't think about individual muscles, we think about whole motions.

The body moves holistically (that is, the body thinks in terms of whole motions). When we move we instinctively and reflexively use our stronger muscles. Also, joints and other ligaments stretch in the direction they are used, and adhesions develop along unused paths of motion. The patterns of strengthening and weakening muscle, as well as the patterns of flexible joints stretching and tight joints restricting, combine to guide the pattern of body motion along a path of least resistance. Just as a piece of paper bends at a fold, over time the tissues of the body literally crease and fold in the way they are used. Body motion follows the folds of our body's functional creases.

In order to stretch a tight muscle, or to fold the body along a different fold of motion, we must restrict the motion of a more mobile, or looser, adjacent joint. Therefore, when restoring motion to the links of a kinetic chain,

Remember:
First: Lock the Stretched Joint,
Then: Stretch the Locked Joint.

THE 4TH POSTURE PRINCIPLE, COMPENSATION (Function)

THE BODY LEARNS TO MOVE IN THE PATTERNS YOU TEACH IT... AND PAIN TEACHES THE BODY TO MOVE DIFFERENTLY

Your unique BodyType, injuries and LifeHabits have trained you to move your body in a unique pattern of motion. Since motion follows the path of least resistance, and pain teaches the body to move in different patterns of motion, when you are injured your body compensates by moving differently.

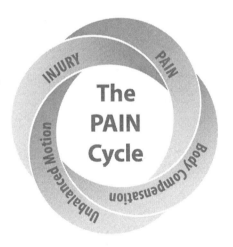

THE PAIN CYCLE
Injury causes pain and tissue damage.
Pain causes the body to compensate.
The body compensates and adapts.
The body moves differently to avoid pain.
Unbalanced Motion and Poor Posture stress muscles and joints, causing injury.

The Pain Cycle begins as functional compensation, and over time progresses to structural adaptation as the body learns to move in pain avoidance patterns. Some muscles become chronically tight and others weaken as injured tissues are avoided. Function, or how we do things, changes. Asymmetric posture and unbalanced or "trick" patterns of motion cause some ligaments to shorten and others to stretch as some joints stiffen and others become unstable.

Whether the cycle begins with unbalanced motion from an injury, or even habitual poor posture, the body compensates for pain by moving differently, compensating and adapting in an ever worsening cycle of poor posture, poor balance, and increased biomechanical stress. As a paper clip bent back and forth weakens at the bend, over time mechanically inefficient patterns of poor posture and unbalanced motion create the PAIN CYCLE, resulting in a continuous loop of increased body stress, joint degeneration (osteoarthritis), chronic pain and recurring injury.

The Pain Cycle of injury-pain-compensation-adaptation creates a vicious cycle of poor posture, adaptive body motion, increased bio-mechanical stress and premature degeneration.

THE 5TH POSTURE PRINCIPLE, ADAPTATION (Structure)

CHANGES IN POSTURE & MOTION CAUSE THE BODY TO CHANGE...FOR BETTER OR FOR WORSE

"A body at rest tends to stay at rest. A body in motion tends to stay in motion" Newton's 1st Law of Motion

Functionally, we know The Body Learns What You Teach It and that Practice makes Permanent, not perfect. The Pain Cycle creates a vicious spiral of compensating posture and adaptive motion because we get better at doing whatever we do. Structurally, the body changes and loses strength, flexibility, and ease of motion.

In other words, we move old.

However, there is hope. If pain is the problem, then motion can be the solution. Since the body adapts to the stresses we place upon it, focused posture exercises can break the Pain Cycle with a virtuous cycle of balanced motion.

The Motion Cycle is the solution for the Pain Cycle's asymmetrical, compensatory poor posture and adaptive body motion patterns. When joints are unlocked to move freely and muscles trained to stabilize through a full range of motion, weak muscles strengthen, adaptively tight muscles stretch, and ligaments adapt in a virtuous cycle of motion.

THE MOTION CYCLE

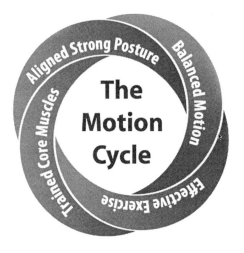

• Stable and StrongPosture™ promotes balanced motion. (StrongPosture™ exercise)
• Balanced and Full Motion allows joints and muscles to move in their normal range. (Spinal Manipulation and Muscle Therapy)
• Normal and balanced motion allows Effective Exercise in an active lifestyle.
• Trained Muscles learn to be strong, flexible and in control for well-balanced, stable posture.

Focused Motion Posture exercises create the Motion Cycle. StrongPosture™ exercises train muscles to be strong, flexible, and in control for well balanced stable posture and ease of motion as you age. Free, balanced motion reduces joint stress, relieves pain, and restores flexibility to break the Pain Cycle.

You use it or lose it. The Goal is Balance, Flexibility & Control. Restoring balanced motion and posture helps restore vitality. The Motion Cycle of strong, stable posture and balanced, flexible motion helps keep the body moving naturally, feeling good, and aging well.

Posture compensation and adaptive motion prematurely age the body. StrongPosture™ and balanced motion keep you moving well as you age.

Have You Done Your StrongPosture™ Exercises Today?

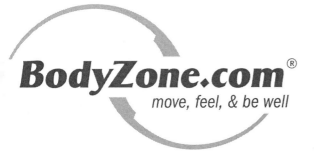

Appendix C: Assessment Form
Download full size version at:
www.posturezone.com/pages/book

Posture Assessment

About your Digital Posture Assessment

Your posture is how you show yourself to the world and how others view you. Besides making you look old before your time, the imbalances and misalignments of chronic poor posture stresses muscles and joints, and the body adapts. Low back and neck pain, headaches, bursitis, arthritis and other structural or mechanical problems may result.

The purpose of this screening is to observe your posture and how your body balances. Exercises and/or strategies to help strengthen your posture may be suggested.

Front Posture Observations
- ☐ Within normal range
- ☐ Postural distortions noted:

Head tilt to	☐ L	☐ R
High shoulder	☐ L	☐ R
Shoulder roll	☐ L	☐ R
Arm away	☐ L	☐ R
Arm long	☐ L	☐ R
Hip high	☐ L	☐ R
Knee roll-in	☐ L	☐ R

  Feet
  -LT ☐ toe in/out ☐ roll in/out
  -RT ☐ toe in/out ☐ roll in/out

Side Posture Observations
- ☐ Within normal range
- ☐ Posture Distortions noted:

  Upper Cross Posture Syndrome
  - ☐ Forward Head Posture (FHP)
  - ☐ Head extension posture
  - ☐ Shoulder girdle roll-in

  Lower Cross Posture Syndrome
  - ☐ Adaptive short hip flexors
  - ☐ Low back hyper-extension
  - ☐ Abdominal protrusion

Suggestions: To keep moving well as you age, remember: **BE POSTURE CONSCIOUS!**

Strong posture is important for good health and aging well. Postural symmetry affects your muscles, joints and overall health. Strong, well-aligned posture minimizes stress and helps reduce pain. Weak posture forces you to work harder to balance as you fight gravity in everything you do, stressing muscles and even prematurely wearing joints (arthritis).

Consider the following StrongPosture LifeHabits:
- ☐ Posture focus with exercise
- ☐ Stork One Leg Balance exercise
- ☐ Read Stand Taller~Live Longer pp._____
- ☐ Stretch the adaptively tight muscle groups noted above
- ☐ Strengthen the adaptively weak muscle groups noted above
- ☐ Consult for stress relief or focused muscle therapy:
- ☐ Consult for a complete biomechanical evaluation:

This assessment is intended to provide you with insight into your posture and body mechanics, and is not intended to diagnose or treat serious neck, back or other spinal conditions.

Any exercises suggested should be reviewed by your healthcare provider to ensure appropriateness for you unique posture and clinical history.

StrongPosture™ Exercise Helps you Move, Feel and Be Well

We are dedicated to teaching people about posture and moving well. Contact us to arrange a posture screening for your organization.

© 2011 BodyZone.com All Rights Reserved. Images courtesy Stand Taller~Live Longer, © Steven Weiniger DC

Appendix C: Posture Zone Assessment Form
Download full size version at:
www.posturezone.com/pages/book

PostureZone.com Assessment

NAME: _____ DATE: _____

	Front View	Back View	Side View
Zone 4: **Head**	**Head Tilt** High R___ L___ Rotation R___ L___ TMJ R___ L___ **Neck………………..** SCM Hypertrophy R___ L___ Short R___ L___ Head Weight Balance ___Aligned ___Forward ___Asymmetric ___Stressed ___Forward ___mild ___mod ___severe	**Head Tilt** High R___ L___ Rotation R___ L___ TMJ Distortion R___ L___ **Neck………………..** SCM Hypertrophy R___ L___ Short R___ L___ Head Weight Balance ___Aligned ___Forward ___Asymmetric ___Stressed ___Forward ___mild ___mod ___severe	**Weight Balance: Head** ___Aligned ___Neutral ___Asymmetric ___Stressed ___Forward - mild ___Forward - moderate ___Forward - severe **Neck………………..** ___Neutral ___Extension adaptation ___Flexion adaptation Cervical Curve ___Normal ___Flat ___Increase
Zone 3: **Torso**	**Chest…………………..** Breathing Pattern ___Neutral ___Chest ___Depressed ___Chest Assist ___Diaphragmatic Weight Balance ___Aligned ___Depressed ___Back Rounded ___Back Flat **Upper Extremity…………….** Clavicular Grooves R___ L___ SHOULDERS ___Aligned ___ Rolled in ___ High on the R___ L___ Short trapezius R___ L___ Short levator scapula R___ L___ **ARMS………………………** ___Aligned ___Forward ___Rolled in Tight arm - Body space R L **HANDS…..** ___Aligned ___Forward ___Bilateral ___Internally Rotated Hand rolled in R___ L___	**Upper Back…………………..** ___Aligned ___Asymmetric ___Stressed ___Rounded ___Flattened Spinal Muscles Hypertrophy R___ L___ Hypotropy R___ L___ **Upper Extremity…………..** SHOULDERS High on the R___ L___ Scapula Winging R___ L___ Scapula Rotation ADDucted R___ L___ ABDucted R___ L___ **ARMS………………………..** Tight arm - Body space R___ L___ **HANDS…..** ___Aligned ___Forward ___Bilateral ___Internally rotated Hand rolled in R___ L___	**Weight Balance:Torso** ___Aligned ___Neutral ___Asymmetric ___Stressed ___Back ___Forward ___Severely Back Torso - Chest ___Neutral ___Back Rounded ___Depressed ___Back Flat **Upper Extremity………..** Shoulders ___Aligned ___Rolled in Arms ___Aligned ___Forward ___Rolled in
Zone 2: **Pelvis**	Abdomen Umilicus ___Centered, Deviated R___ L___ Pelvis ___Aligned Drop - High on R___ L___ Rotation R back ___ L back ___	Low Back Mid-back spinal muscles Hypertrophy R___ L___ Hypotropy R___ L___ Lumbar crease noted on the R___ L___ Low-back spinal muscles Hypertrophy R___ L___ Hypotropy R___ L___ Pelvis……. ___ Aligned………… Drop - High on R___ L___ Rotation R back ___ L back ___	**Weight Balance:Pelvis** ___Aligned ___Neutral ___Asymmetric ___Stressed ___Back ___Forward **Low Back…………….** ___Aligned ___Asymmetric ___Stressed ___Flattened ___Mild Arc ___Moderate Arch ___Severe Arch **Abdomen…** ___Aligned……. ___Protruding Pelvic Tilt ___Forward ___Back
Zone 1: **Lower Extremity**	___LE Aligned ___Asymmetric IT Band Groove R___ L___ **Knees…………** ___Neut ___Hyper-ext ___Asymmetric LT: RT: ___Int ___Ext ___Int ___Ext ___Hyp-ext ___Flex ___Hyp-ext ___Flex ___Valga ___Vara ___Valga ___Vara **FEET** ___Symmetric ___Asymmetric **LT Foot** ___Neut. ___Turned out ___Pronate ___Supinat ___Clench ___Hammer **RT Foot** ___Neut. ___Turned out ___Pronate ___Supinat ___Clench ___Hammer	Wt Balance ___Aligned ___Asymmetric IT Band Groove R___ L___ **Knees…………** ___Neut ___Hyper-ext ___Asymmetric LT: RT: ___Int ___Ext ___Int ___Ext ___Hyp-ext ___Flex ___Hyp-ext ___Flex ___Valga ___Vara ___Valga ___Vara **FEET** ___Symmetric ___Asymmetric **LT Foot** ___Neut. ___Turned out ___Pronate ___Supinat ___Clench ___Hammer **RT Foot** ___Neut. ___Turned out ___Pronate ___Supinat ___Clench ___Hammer	**Weight Balance: LE** ___Aligned ___Neutral ___Asymmetric ___Stressed ___Back ___Forward **Knees…….** ___Neutral ___Hyper-extended ___Asymmetric

© 2011 BodyZone.com All Rights Reserved 770-922-0700

Appendix D: Posture Assessment Intake Form
Download customizable version at:
www.posturezone.com/pages/book

Posture Assessment Form

The purpose of this screening is to observe your posture, how you stand and how you balance.
(*Posture is HOW you Balance your body – The 2nd Posture Principle*)
Exercises and/or strategies to help strengthen your posture may be suggested.

1. My general fitness level is

   0   2   4   6   8   10
   (sedentary) (light exercise) (moderate exercise) (athletic)

2. Please note areas where you have experienced pain, stiffness or numbness in the last 6 months.

   2a. Please circle the area of worst pain and mark how bad it is on a scale of 1-10, 10 being severe pain.

   0   1   2   3   4   5   6   7   8   9   10
   No Pain   Severe Pain

   2b. Please note other structural/bio-mechanical problems:

   ___ Headaches   ___ Fatigue
   ___ Arthritis   ___ Stiffness
   ___ Muscle spasm
   ___ Other injuries (auto accidents, sports injuries etc) *describe*:
   _____

3. Do you have any other medical conditions? ___NO ___YES*
   **IF YES, Please describe on reverse*

Office Use   Initials _____
- ☐Y ☐N Hx/ Surg/ Med   ☐Y ☐N Arthritis
- ☐Y ☐N HiBP/Circ/Vein   ☐ DC ☐ MA Hx
- ☐Y ☐N Diabetes/PG   ☐ Post ☐ AA ☐ Rx

Name_____ Email_____

Occupation_____ Age_____ Phone_____

Address_____ City_____ State___ Zip_____

☐ Please subscribe me to your newsletter. *We respect your privacy and will never share your email.*

Posture Assessment Release
It is my choice to have my posture checked. I acknowledge that this evaluation is educational only, and that a thorough in-office examination by a qualified healthcare provider is required for clinical examination or diagnosis. I have stated all medical conditions of which I am aware and I hereby release this practice and professional from any consequences of this evaluation.

SIGNATURE: _____

DATE: _____

© 2011 BodyZone.com All Rights Reserved. Images courtesy Stand Taller~Live Longer, Steven Weiniger DC

Resources

Hot links to these resources and more online at:
www.PostureZone.com/pages/resources

Posture Science & Research

Scoliosis
About: http://www.ncbi.nlm.nih.gov/pubmedhealth/PMH0002221/
Forward bend test: http://www.ncbi.nlm.nih.gov/pubmedhealth/PMH0002221/figure/A001241.B19465/
Spinal curves: http://www.ncbi.nlm.nih.gov/pubmedhealth/PMH0002221/figure/A001241.B19463
Postural Instability in Early-Stage Idiopathic Scoliosis in Adolescent Girls
http://journals.lww.com/spinejournal/Fulltext/2011/06010/Postural_Instability_in_Early_Stage_Idiopathic.17.aspx

Parkinson's Disease
http://www.gaitposture.com/article/S0966-6362(07)00141-5/abstract

Posture and Falls
Fall Prevention: http://www.fallprevention.ri.gov/Module3/sld001.htm
Gait characteristics of elderly people with a history of falls: a dynamic approach. http://www.ncbi.nlm.nih.gov/pubmed/17079750
Quantitative assessment of posture stability using computerized dynamic posturography in type 2 diabetic patients with neuropathy. http://www.ncbi.nlm.nih.gov/pubmed/19551316

Anatomy
http://www.emory.edu/ANATOMY/AnatomyManual/back.html
http://www.getbodysmart.com/

Clinical Posture
Forward head posture: http://www.ncbi.nlm.nih.gov/pubmed/17595423
Posture and Lung Capacity http://www.archives-pmr.org/article/S0003-9993(05)01472-3/abstract
Chiropractic and Posture, Immediate Effects of Lumbar Spine Manipulation on the Resting and Contraction Thickness of Transversus Abdominis in Asymptomatic Individuals http://www.ncbi.nlm.nih.gov/pubmed/20972346
Reflex control of the spine and posture: a review of the literature from a chiropractic perspective. http://www.ncbi.nlm.nih.gov/pubmed/16091134
Massage and Posture: https://www2.uwstout.edu/news/index.asp?event=news.get&ID=2007
Pilates and Posture http://www.ncbi.nlm.nih.gov/pubmed/19404180
Yoga and Posture: http://www.ncbi.nlm.nih.gov/pmc/articles/PMC1447294/
Alexander Technique and Posture: http://www.ncbi.nlm.nih.gov/pubmed/15921477

Posture Assessment
The reliability of quantifying upright standing postures as a baseline diagnostic clinical tool: http://www.ncbi.nlm.nih.gov/entrez/query.fcgi?cmd=Retrieve&db=pubmed&dopt=Citation&list_uids=14970809
Repeatability over time of posture, radiograph positioning, and radiograph line drawing: an analysis of six control groups. http://www.ncbi.nlm.nih.gov/pubmed/12584507
Influence of posture on the range of axial rotation and coupled lateral flexion of the thoracic spine http://www.ncbi.nlm.nih.gov/entrez/query.fcgi?db=pubmed&cmd=Retrieve&dopt=Citation&list_uids=17416273

Posture and Blood Pressure
The Neurochemically Diverse Intermedius Nucleus of the Medulla as a Source of Excitatory and Inhibitory Synaptic Input to the Nucleus Tractus Solitarii http://www.jneurosci.org/content/27/31/8324.abstract

Sitting Postures:
Sitting posture of subjects with postural backache.
http://www.ncbi.nlm.nih.gov/pubmed/16584946
Desk Chairs That Make You Healthier
http://allforhealthcare.blogspot.com/2011/05/desk-chairs-that-make-you-healthier.html?spref=tw
Balanced sitting posture on forward sloping seat
http://www.bodyzone.com/site/body-lifehabits/best-way-to-sit-tilt-the-seat-forward-sitting-postures.html

Posture and Breathing
Why Sucking In Your Stomach Harms Your Health http://www.bottomlinesecrets.com/article.html?article_id=100003061
Effects of an exercise program on respiratory function, posture and on quality of life in osteoporotic women: a pilot study http://www.sciencedirect.com
Impaired postural compensation for respiration in people with recurrent low back pain. http://www.ncbi.nlm.nih.gov/pubmed/12759796
Coexistence of stability and mobility in postural control: evidence from postural compensation for respiration. http://www.ncbi.nlm.nih.gov/pubmed/12021811
Effect of body posture on respiratory impedance.
http://www.ncbi.nlm.nih.gov/pubmed/3356637
Influence of posture on mechanical parameters derived from respiratory impedance. http://www.ncbi.nlm.nih.gov/pubmed/1426223
Effects of posture on the coordination of respiration and swallowing. http://www.ncbi.nlm.nih.gov/pubmed/7884469

Posture Education

Posture Professional referral directory
http://www.bodyzone.com/site/posture-pro-locator/search.html

Patient and Client Education on posture, health and fitness.
http://www.BodyZone.com

History of Good Posture
Teaching Good Posture - 1920's http://video.google.com/videoplay?docid=3777523842754521258&q=1920+posture&total=7&start=0&num=10&so=0&type=search&plindex=1
Posture Class, High School – 1930's
http://www.youtube.com/watch?v=0orvjDvZMCA
A Vintage Guide to Good Posture - 1940's
http://www.youtube.com/watch?v=rbFymPk1FyE
Posture Habits (Highlights) – 1950's
http://www.youtube.com/watch?v=JCmjfjKj9Mo

Professional Tools

Posture Assessment: Grids, analysis software, books and forms, community lectures, screening banners, patient/client education handouts, posters, posture correction protocols, professional tools and equipment.
http://www.PostureZone.com   1-866-443-8966

Professional Training

Posture Exercise Professional Certification (CPEP) StrongPosture™ Exercise Protocols: Posture Practice implementation and posture assessment presented as continuing education approved seminars, live workshops, keynotes and on-site group training, as well as, online video-based courses, webinars and teleconferences.
http://www.PosturePractice.com   770-922-0700

Speaker / Instructor Information
http://www.standtallerlivelonger.com

Social Media – Professional Posture Updates
http://twitter.com/posturezone
http://facebook.com/posturezone

Sources

Stand Taller ~ Live Longer: An Anti-Aging Strategy, Steven Weiniger, DC, BodyZone.com Press, 2008

StrongPosture™ Exercise Professional Training Manual, Steven Weiniger, DC, BodyZone.com Press, 2005, 2011

Posture Pictures: A tool for building a Patient Choice Practice, Steven Weiniger, DC, BodyZone.com Press, 2007

The Five Posture Principles, Steven Weiniger, DC, BodyZone.com Press, 2005

(Endnotes)

1. *Posture Pictures: A tool for building a Patient Choice Practice, Steven Weiniger, DC, BodyZone.com Press, 2007*

2. *How Doctors Think, Jerome Groopman, Houghton Mifflin Company 2007*

3. *Harvard Medical School Adviser, Harvard Publishing, January 24, 2006*

4. *Height Loss in Older Men- Associations With Total Mortality and Incidence of Cardiovascular Disease S. Goya Wannamethee, PhD; A. Gerald*

5. *Hyperkyphotic posture predicts mortality in older community-dwelling men and women: a prospective study, D. Kado, MD, Huang, DrPH, A. Karlamangla, MD, PhD*, et.al., Journal of the American Geriatrics Society, Volume 52 issue10, p1662 -10/2004*

6. *The Five Posture Principles, Steven Weiniger, DC, BodyZone.com Press, 2005*

7. *Muscles: Testing and Function, with Posture and Pain, Kendall & McCreary Lippincott Williams & Wilkins; Fifth, North American Edition edition (February 24, 2005)*

8. *Rehabilitation of the Spine: A Practitioner's Manual, Craig Liebenson, Lippincott Williams & Wilkins, 2006*

9. *Structural yoga therapy, Mukunda Stiles, 2000, Red Wheel Weiser, San Francisco, CA*

10. *Egoscue Posture Solutions, Pete Egoscue*

11. *Stand Taller ~ Live Longer: An Anti-Aging Strategy, Steven Weiniger, DC, BodyZone.com Press, 2008*

12. *Postural Assessment Chapter 2, Steven Weiniger, DC in Photographic Manual of Regional Orthopaedic and Neurological tests, 4th ed, Cipriano, J, Lippincott Williams & Wilkins 2003*

13. *StrongPosture™ Exercise Professional Training Manual, Steven Weiniger, DC, BodyZone.com Press, 2005, 2011*

14. *Implications for the use of postural analysis as a clinical diagnostic tool: Reliability of quantifying upright standing spinal postures from photographic images, DunkM; LaLonde J; Callaghan, J of manipulative and physiological therapeutics 2005, vol. 28, no8, pp. 386-392*

Certified Posture Exercise Professional - CPEP
Program for Health & Fitness Professionals

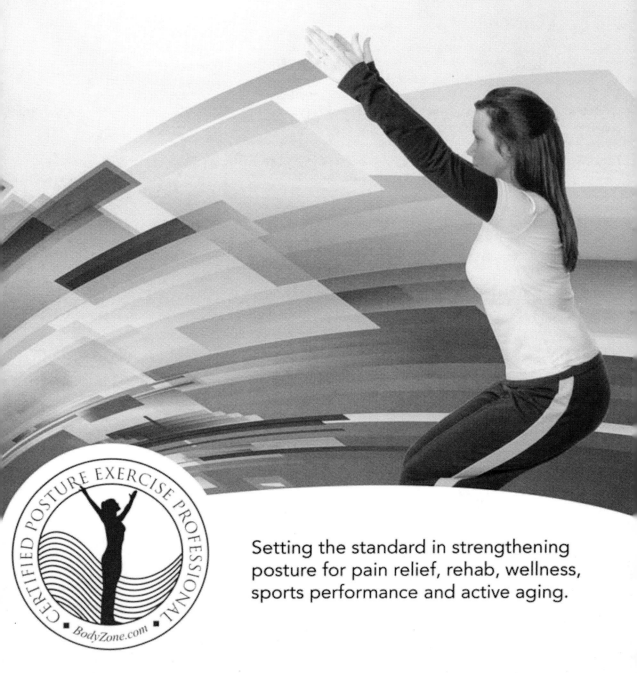

Setting the standard in strengthening posture for pain relief, rehab, wellness, sports performance and active aging.

CPEP PROGRAM

Want to help more people move well? Join the international network of Certified Posture Exercise Professionals (CPEP).

CPEPs are independent health and fitness professionals trained in StrongPosture™ exercise protocols, and have demonstrated proficiency in teaching and adapting the protocols to people of various levels of fitness and ability.

Posture is the "Function of Structure" and this research documented course will teach you to assess, communicate and strengthen posture. Back pain and other neuromusculoskeletal conditions result from weak posture, and strengthening structural balance and functional alignment helps relieve pain, optimize sports performance, improve appearance and promote successful aging.

Put simply, this "step it up" program is for professionals who want to position themselves as the local posture expert. Professionals can take their practices to the next level with CPEP certification and perfect a bio-mechanical model that teaches focused motion exercise as integral to strengthening posture while improving balance and function.

"My patients see immediate results themsel
it's easy, and th

EDUCATIONAL OVERVIEW

StrongPosture™ exercise protocols build a road to a successful practice which integrates active and passive care for improved results, referrals and retention.

Participants learn strategies to build the three dimensions of a Posture Practice:

BodyZone.co
move, feel, & be

Posture **Consciousness**

- Creating awareness of posture perception vs. reality
- Assessing standing posture and gait biomechanics
- Building a structural baseline with annual posture pictures
- Training people to become more "posture-conscious" during daily activity

Posture **Concepts**

- Why "perfect posture" is a myth
- Assessments by PostureZone for Upper and Lower Cross syndromes
- Balance, Alignment and Motion: the three elements of posture
- 5 Posture Principles for teaching patient-friendly biomechanics
- Communications that target common complaints including: back pain, computer workers with forward head posture, teens with rolled in shoulders, athletes seeking biomechanical efficiency, and the growing market niche of Boomers and seniors

Posture **Control**

- Individualized focused-motion exercises progress along three tracks: Balance, Alignment and Motion
- Protocols to strengthen control of alignment and motion of the pelvis, head, and torso
- Recognizing and correcting abnormal muscle patterns
- Retrain deep core muscle recruitment towards symmetric motion with balls, bands, foam and other tools
- Engaging forgotten motion patterns to target weak kinetic links for pain management, rehab and improved posture

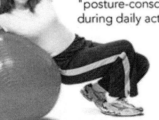

WHO IS ELIGIBLE TO ENROLL?

Doctors (DC, MD, DO, DPM, etc.), therapists (MT, PT, OT), physicians assistants, chiropractic therapy assistants, athletic and personal trainers, coaches, nurses, senior care specialists, yoga and Pilates instructors, as well as other health and fitness professionals.

www.PosturePractice.com
770-922-0700

IS IT RIGHT FOR MY CLIENTS/PATIENTS?

Teen to Boomer, pregnant to elderly, athlete to desperately deconditioned, posture exercise is applicable to just about every lifestyle, age, and fitness level.

Whether a patient/client is recovering from an injury or preparing for the Olympics, the protocol can be customized to fit their specific needs.

HOW WILL CPEP FIT MY PRACTICE?

StrongPosture™ protocols are a framework - or flow of exercise - you teach a step at a time. Quickly modify exercises for the condition and goal of each individual with 'peelbacks' and 'progressions'. The systematized program is designed to mesh with techniques, therapies and exercises you already offer in practice.

hey feel better immediately; st love to do it." - Dr. Anita Kelley-Dukes

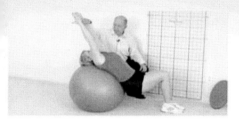 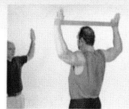 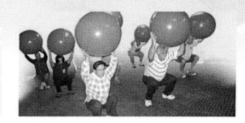

Through the video series, 15 weeks to a Posture Practice, learn a systematic approach to building a PosturePractice and branding yourself as the local 'Posture Expert'.

Week by week you and your team will learn how to confidently communicate StrongPosture™ concepts and teach protocols that engage clients and patients. Materials for successful implementation, marketing and community branding, as well as weekly in-office signage are included.

MARKETING A POSTURE PRACTICE

The branding and marketing component of certification targets your practice's three concentric Circles of Social Influence by focusing on Practice Management, Implementation and Branding.

Management
- Staff training
- In-office changes
- Teaching patients/clients
- Tracking progress and compliance

Implementation
- Patient/client education tools
- Scripting posture communications
- Recalls for retention
- Program design

Branding
- Media releases /Marketing
- Posture assessment and screenings
- Community classes / corporate talks
- Finances

CPEP CERTIFICATION CHECKLIST

PROTOCOL TRAINING

- ☐ Live Posture Practice seminar
  (or train via interactive online platform).
  *Onsite training available for groups, hospitals and educational institutions.

  Online Classes
- ☐ Rehab of Motion & Balance (3hrs)
- ☐ Motion Patterns (3hrs)
- ☐ Compensation & Stabilization (3hrs)
- ☐ Adaptation & Core Retraining (3hrs)
- ☐ StrongPosture & Wellness (3hrs)

  Assessment
- ☐ Written evaluation (online)
- ☐ Practical proficiency (live or online platform, includes review materials and proficiency assessment coaching)

MARKETING TRAINING

- ☐ 15 Weeks to a Posture Practice Video Series
- ☐ Management, Implementation and Branding
- ☐ Implementation forms and marketing materials

POSTURE PRACTICE TOOLS

- ☐ Posture Rehab Protocol Set, includes;
  - Customizable exercise handouts (CD)
  - CPEP Professional Training Manual
  - Balance and Alignment Instructional Video (DVD)
- ☐ PostureZone Assessment Grid
- ☐ Stand Taller ~ Live Longer- (ISBN 0979713609)
- ☐ Posture Pictures: Assessment, Screenings, Marketing & Forms - (ISBN 0979713617)
- ☐ Stand Taller Community Lecture (PowerPoint)

Info, FAQs and Recent Media
www.PosturePractice.com

Ready to Enroll? Questions?
CPEP@BodyZone.com
1-866-443-8966
770-922-0700

PRACTICE BENEFITS

- Implement step-by-step protocols into practice as you
- Progressive sequence takes the guesswork out of ' comes next'
- Posture assessment and balance exam procedures
- Common posture adaptations and distortions
- Research supported active care rehab
- Customize exercises for any body type or ability level
- Offer individualized programs or group classes
- Fast results lead to retention and enthusiastic refe
- Included instructional handouts boost compliance
- Forms for staff training, tracking progress and asses
- Flyers for client/patient education and practice pron
- Feel the difference in your own body as you build StrongPosture™
- Renewed enthusiasm for your practice
- Become the "posture expert" in your community

PATIENT/CLIENT BENEFITS

- Injury rehabilitation
- Improve posture and balance
- Increased mobility and flexibility
- Fluidity of motion
- Enhanced sports performance
- Active aging concepts for longevity
- Easy to remember, step-by-step, program
- Dynamic self-help concepts can be practiced at ho
- Incorporates fun, inexpensive tools

UPON COMPLETION

- CPEP Certificate for display
- CPEP logo for marketing
- CPEP decal for office or vehicle visibility
- BodyZone.com news release to media in your area
- Preferred posture professional locator listing

ONGOING SUPPORT

- BodyZone.com promotes Certified Posture Exerci Professionals (CPEPs) internationally. StrongPostu Exercises and concepts are featured regularly in news
- Participants have access to staff by phone and email for support and program questions.
- CPEP monthly e-newsletter with printable patient education sign, protocol refreshers, posture medi current posture research.
- CPEPs are invited to supplemental training, via live seminars, interactive webinars, and videos posted CPEP resource area.
- CPEP discount on all PostureZone.com tools.

© 2013 BodyZone, LLC All Rights Reserved.

About the Authors

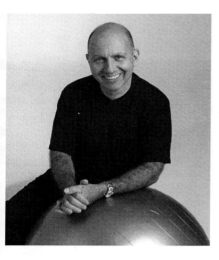

Dr. Steven Weiniger, internationally recognized speaker and posture expert, has trained thousands of doctors, trainers, therapists and other health professionals to rehab injuries and help their patients / clients keep moving well as they age with StrongPosture™ exercise protocols.

His popular seminars including, *Clinical Posture Assessment, Therapy & Exercise* and *Posture Practice*, are hosted by educational, clinical and professional associations in the US and Canada.

He is also lead instructor for the Certified Posture Exercise Professional (CPEP) program. This certification course is creating a network of posture experts. CPEPs are setting a new standard for wellness and anti-aging care in the community.

Dr. Weiniger literally wrote the book about improving posture, *Stand Taller ~ Live Longer: An Anti-Aging Strategy*. He also authored the Postural Assessment chapter in the textbook, Photographic Manual of Regional Orthopedic and Neurological Tests. His articles and expertise on posture, anti-aging, exercise, and practice management have been featured by national media including, industry journals, FOX News, Oprah's Oxygen network, Scripps Howard News, 'Health on the Hill', the publication for the House Committee on Health Care, American Fitness, Bottom Line Personal, Best Self Magazine, Bottom Line Health and most recently, Oxygen Magazine.

An appointed delegate to the White House Conference on Aging (WHCoA), the decennial event held by the President of the United States and Congress, Dr. Weiniger worked with other leaders to develop recommendations on issues, policy and research in the field of aging.

Dr. Steven Weiniger presents lectures for professional organizations internationally and is also continuing education instructor for Logan College of Chiropractic. He's been a featured speaker for many institutions including Northwestern University of Health Sciences, University of Bridgeport Chiropractic College, Association for Health, Physical Education, Recreation & Dance (IAHPERD), Atlanta School of Massage, NCLC, COCSA, Parker Seminars, Palmer College, Dekalb College & Clayton University.

He currently serves as Managing Partner of BodyZone.com, an online resource offering a referral directory and comprehensive information about posture, exercise and other intelligent habits for an active life.

Dr. Weiniger focuses on posture rehab and biomechanics in Atlanta, Georgia. He and his wife enjoy an active lifestyle which includes recumbent cycling, kayaking, skiing, tennis and yoga.

Contact Dr. Steven Weiniger: drw@bodyzone.com   www.PosturePractice.com

- facebook.com/steven.weiniger
- facebook.com/standtaller
- twitter.com/bodyzone
- linkedin.com/in/posture
- youtube.com/postureexercise

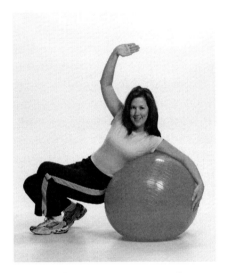

Renée North, CPEP, is Vice President of Operations for BodyZone.com. She is also Master Trainer for the Certified Posture Exercise Professional program, certifying health and fitness professionals in StrongPosture protocols for injury rehab, wellness, sports performance and anti-aging. Renée works with doctors, therapists and trainers to integrate exercise protocols into their practices that are integral to strengthening posture while improving balance, function and activity with patients and clients.

Her articles focusing on positive psychology and the science of happiness as well as health and active aging strategies for all age groups appear in publications worldwide.

Renee also maintains certifications as a Personal Trainer (NASM-CPT) and Pilates Instructor.

- facebook.com/reneenorthcpep
- facebook.com/ PostureZone
- twitter.com/reneenorth
- linkedin.com/in/reneenorth
- youtube.com/happyrenee1

Also available from

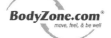

BodyZone Press

Stand Taller ~ Live Longer
An Anti-Aging Strategy

Stand Taller ~ Live Longer: An Anti-Aging Strategy shows healthcare and fitness professionals how to progressively build daily posture exercise routines for the individuals they serve.

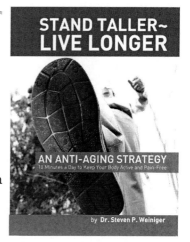

In the process, clients reach a variety of crucial goals:

- Improving posture
- Rehab after injury
- Enhancing sports performance
- Increasing and maintaining activity within the aging population
- Correcting and strengthening posture in everyone from computer-bound teenagers to baby boomers and beyond
- Eliminating pain
- Increasing flexibility

The 7-week program detailed in Stand Taller ~ Live Longer combines cutting-edge research with interactive demonstrations and embodies the philosophy "Use it to keep it." This user friendly program takes just 10 minutes a day and the response, notes the author, Dr. Weiniger, "has been amazing."

He comments, "Doctors, therapists, trainers, instructors, rehab centers, nursing homes, and people in physical education and college athletic departments are using the book to make a significant difference in the lives of those they work with."

Available at www.PostureZone.com.

PostureZone® Has a FREE App
StrongPosture™ begins with an assessment

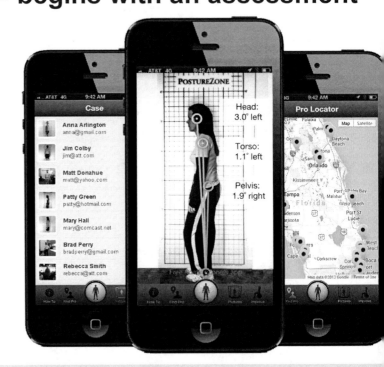

With This App you Can:

- **Reveal subtle imbalances** and asymmetries
- **Set a benchmark** for improving posture
- **Measure changes** in head, torso and pelvis alignment
- **Track and compare** assessments
- **Share posture pictures** on Facebook and Twitter
- **Provide a fast analysis** absolutely anywhere

PostureZone® screenings measure distortions in degrees to clearly identify symmetry, balance, improvements or changes. Quickly observe deviations of misalignment between the head, torso, and pelvis over the center of the feet.

More app features:

- Integrated level ensures accuracy
- Track assessments in pictures gallery
- Regular posture checks build awareness
- Analyze front, side and back views
- Measure changes in head, torso and pelvis alignment

Are you a professional?

PostureZone features **Find Pro** directory making it easy for users to find a local posture professional. To get listed visit: *www.StrongPosture.com/support*

Optional one time in-app purchase of PostureZone Pro adds case management tap to zoom, additional export options via iTunes & email, PosturePractice videos, w no monthly or usage fees.

To learn more, scan the barcode or visit us at www.StrongPosture.com

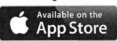

Brought to you by:

  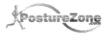 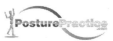

© 2013 BodyZone, LLC All Rights Reserved